THE SMALL BUT MIGHTY THYROID

MEET YOUR TINY QUEEN OF HEALTH AND ENERGY

TIFFANY ROSE

CONTENTS

INTRODUCTION

Meet Jessica. Jessica is a 40-something woman who juggles work, family, and the occasional girls' night out. She's a superhero in her own right, but lately, Jessica has been feeling less like Wonder Woman and more like a wilted houseplant. She's always tired, her hair is thinning, and she's gained a few stubborn pounds that refuse to budge. After months of frustration and confusion, Jessica finally visits her Doctor, only to be told, "It's just stress. Your labs came back all within normal range." Sound familiar?

Hi, I'm Tiffany Rose, and my passion for this topic is deeply personal. For years, I struggled to understand what was happening to me. I used to be the queen of time management and to-do lists, always on top of things. Then, slowly, my energy began to fade. At first, I brushed it off as just getting older. But the occasional fatigue became chronic; my clothes didn't fit the same, and my hair started thinning. I became intolerant to cold, and my quality of life declined. It was clear that something was going on with my body—it wasn't just aging.

After being told multiple times that all my blood work had come back normal, I was feeling frustrated and confused. Desperate for answers, I began researching my symptoms, and I started suspecting my thyroid might be the issue—something I'd heard about but never imagined would affect me. I then started asking my doctor to check my thyroid, still not knowing anything about the thyroid, except I knew I had some symptoms. Despite repeatedly asking my doctor to test my thyroid, the results always came back 'normal,' and my concerns were dismissed. Like many, I thought 'normal' lab results meant everything was fine. But I was wrong.

I felt lost trying to navigate my symptoms within today's medical system. I was stuck, feeling miserable, and drained of energy and motivation. Anxiety constantly loomed in the background, and I no longer felt in control of my health. I refused to accept that this was my new normal. Determined to find answers, I heard about Functional Medicine Doctors and their approach to addressing the root causes of symptoms rather than just treating them. I felt a glimmer of hope again.

I know firsthand how a small gland in your neck can disrupt your life. However, I also understand how gaining knowledge and taking control of your thyroid health can transform your quality of life, allowing you to thrive—even if medication becomes part of your daily routine. I've learned a great deal about the thyroid, and I want to share this knowledge with women around the world who are seeking answers like I was when our doctors told us that our blood work is "within the normal range."

The purpose of this book is simple: to be your trusty guide through the maze of thyroid health. We'll cover everything from understanding thyroid hormones to recognizing symptoms and discussing natural remedies. Think of it as your thyroid's owner's manual, with a sprinkle of humor and a lot of heart.

Why is thyroid health so important? The thyroid gland may be small, but it's mighty. It controls your metabolism, energy levels, and even your mood. When it's not working right, you're not working right. Picture your thyroid as the queen of your body's hormonal kingdom. When the queen is unhappy, the entire realm is in chaos.

Women, especially those in perimenopause, often face unique challenges when it comes to thyroid health. Symptoms like fatigue, weight gain, and mood swings are frequently brushed off as "just part of aging." But you deserve better than that. You deserve to feel energetic, vibrant, and in control.

In this book, we'll explore lifestyle changes that can support your thyroid. From diet tweaks to stress management techniques, you'll find practical advice you can start using today. We'll also discuss the importance of gut health, the pituitary gland's role, and how toxins affect your thyroid.

Knowledge is power. When it comes to your health, being informed is the first step to feeling better. This book aims to give you the information you need to make educated decisions. We'll dive into the details of thyroid blood panels so you know what to ask your Doctor. We'll also discuss the nuances of Hashimoto's disease and hyperthyroidism so you can understand what's really going on in your body.

So, dear reader, are you ready to take control of your thyroid health? This book is your roadmap. Together, we'll navigate the twists and turns, with a few laughs along the way, and empower you to feel like the queen you are.

Your Friend,

Tiffany Rose

1

THYROID BASICS: UNDERSTANDING YOUR TINY QUEEN

One day, while sipping her third cup of coffee and trying to summon the energy for a full day of meetings, Sarah suddenly felt a wave of exhaustion wash over her. This wasn't the usual tiredness from a late night or an early morning. No, this bone-deep fatigue made her feel like she was wading through molasses. After weeks of feeling off, she finally decided to visit her doctor, who suggested checking her thyroid. Little did Sarah know, this tiny gland was about to explain so much about her recent struggles.

You might be wondering why a small gland in your neck can have such a profound effect on your life. Let's get to know the thyroid, your tiny queen of health and energy. This chapter will be your introduction to this powerful little gland, setting the stage for everything we'll cover in the book.

THE QUEEN OF METABOLISM: WHAT IS THE THYROID?

The thyroid is a butterfly-shaped gland located at the base of your neck, just below your Adam's apple. Despite its small size, it's a critical part of your endocrine system, the network of glands that produce and regulate hormones. Imagine it as the queen of your internal kingdom, ruling over your metabolism with an iron fist. When the queen is unhappy, the entire realm suffers.

Historically, the thyroid has fascinated medical practitioners for centuries. Ancient Greek physicians, like Hippocrates and Galen, mentioned the thyroid in their work. They recognized its importance, even if they didn't fully understand it. In ancient Greece, the neck and throat were often seen as symbols of strength and vulnerability. The thyroid, nestled in this crucial area, was believed to hold the key to vitality and health. This belief has carried through the ages, and modern science has only deepened our understanding of its significance.

Now, let's talk about why the thyroid is often called the "Queen of Metabolism." This gland produces hormones controlling your metabolic rate, which is how fast or slow your body converts food into energy. When your thyroid functions properly, it helps maintain a balanced metabolism, ensuring you have enough energy to get through your day without feeling like a zombie. It also plays a crucial role in weight management. If your thyroid is underactive (hypothyroidism), you might struggle with weight gain. On the flip side, an overactive thyroid (hyperthyroidism) can lead to weight loss and an increased appetite.

To understand how it all works, we need a quick anatomy and physiology lesson. The thyroid is made up of tiny sacs called follicles, which store a protein called thyroglobulin. This protein is crucial for the production of thyroid hormones. The two main hormones produced by the thyroid are T3 (triiodothyronine) and T4 (thyroxine). These hormones are released into the bloodstream and travel to various tissues in your body, regulating metabolism and energy levels.

But the thyroid doesn't work alone. It takes its orders from the pituitary gland, a tiny pea-sized gland located at the base of your brain. The pituitary gland produces thyroid-stimulating hormone (TSH), which signals the thyroid to produce and release T3 and T4. Think of TSH as the royal advisor, whispering instructions to the queen on how to keep the kingdom running smoothly.

When everything is balanced, your thyroid and pituitary gland work together like a well-oiled machine. But when things go awry, it can lead to many issues. An underactive thyroid can cause symptoms like fatigue, weight gain, and depression. An overactive thyroid, on the other hand, can result in anxiety, weight loss, and palpitations.

Understanding the basics of your thyroid is the first step in taking control of your health. In the following chapters, we'll dig deeper into the specifics of thyroid hormones, common disorders, and how you can support your thyroid naturally. But for now, remember that your thyroid, though small, is mighty. It's the queen of your metabolism, and keeping her happy is key to feeling your best.

THYROID HORMONES: THE ROYAL MESSENGERS

Let's talk about the thyroid hormones, the royal messengers of your body. These are not just any ordinary hormones; they are the VIPs of your endocrine system. The two main players here are Triiodothyronine (T3) and Thyroxine (T4). Think of T4 as the queen's envoy, traveling far and wide, while T3 is the queen's secret weapon, delivering the final, powerful punch. T4 is produced in larger quantities but is less potent. It's like a diplomat who needs to be converted into a more effective agent—T3— before making a real impact.

The production and secretion of these hormones are fascinating processes. Your thyroid gland relies heavily on iodine, a mineral found in foods like fish, dairy, and iodized salt. Iodine is the raw material your thyroid uses to produce T4 and T3. Imagine iodine as the fabric for the queen's royal robes. Without it, she's got nothing to wear! Once the thyroid captures iodine from your bloodstream, it combines it with tyrosine, an amino acid, to create T4 and T3. T4 then gets converted to T3 in various tissues throughout your body, like the liver and kidneys. This conversion is crucial because T3 is the more active form, the one that truly gets things done.

So, how do these royal messengers interact with your body? When T3 and T4 are released into your bloodstream, they travel to cells and bind to thyroid hormone receptors. This binding process is akin to the queen's envoys delivering messages to the lords and ladies of the realm. Once they latch onto these receptors, they regulate gene expression, which means they can turn certain genes on or off. This regulation is vital for protein synthesis, influencing how your body repairs itself, grows, and maintains its myriad functions.

The systemic effects of these hormones are wide-ranging and incredibly impactful. In the cardiovascular system, T3 and T4 help regulate heart rate and blood pressure. If you've ever felt your heart race or slow down inexplicably, your thyroid might be playing a role. For the digestive system, these hormones control your metabolic rate, affecting how efficiently you digest food and absorb nutrients. Have you ever wondered why some people seem to eat anything without gaining weight while others struggle? Your thyroid could be the key.

Regarding the nervous system, thyroid hormones are essential for cognitive function and mood regulation. Ever experienced brain fog or a sudden bout of irritability? That might be your thyroid acting up. These hormones ensure that your neurons fire correctly and that neurotransmitters, the chemicals responsible for mood, are in balance. Their influence extends to virtually every part of your body, making them indispensable for overall well-being.

To bring this all home, let's consider a real-life example. Imagine you're preparing for a big presentation at work. You've got your notes, your slides, and your outfit ready. But on the morning of the presentation, you wake up feeling groggy, your heart is racing, and you can't seem to focus. You haven't changed your routine, so what gives? Your thyroid hormones might be out of whack, causing a cascade of symptoms that throw your whole day off.

Understanding how these hormones work and their far-reaching effects can empower you to take control of your health. Whether it's tweaking your diet to include more iodine-rich foods or discussing hormone replacement therapy with your doctor, knowing the role of T3 and T4 gives you the tools to make informed decisions.

In this chapter, we've explored the majestic world of thyroid hormones, those royal messengers that keep your body in balance. They might be small molecules, but their impact is monumental. They regulate your metabolism, influence your heart and digestive systems, and affect your mood and cognitive function. So, next time you feel off, remember that it could be your thyroid's royal messengers trying to send you a signal.

THE THYROID AND YOUR BODY: A SYMBIOTIC RELATIONSHIP

Imagine your body as a bustling city with various departments working together to keep things running smoothly. Your thyroid is like the city's power plant, providing energy and regulating the flow of resources. But it doesn't work in isolation. It's part of a complex network of glands, each playing a crucial role. One of the key players in this network is the pituitary gland. Often referred to as the "master gland," the pituitary is like the city's central command center. It releases thyroid-stimulating hormone (TSH), which tells the thyroid when to produce more hormones. Without these orders, your thyroid wouldn't know how much T3 and T4 to pump out, leading to chaos in your body's systems.

Another vital gland in this network is the adrenal gland. These sit atop your kidneys and are responsible for producing stress hormones like cortisol. When you're stressed, your adrenal glands go into overdrive, releasing cortisol to help you cope. But chronic stress can throw a wrench into the works. High cortisol levels can interfere with the conversion of T4 to T3, leading to a sluggish thyroid. It's like having a power outage in your city because the emergency services are stretched too thin. This is why managing stress is so essential for maintaining thyroid health.

Beyond its role in metabolism, your thyroid influences several major bodily functions. For starters, it plays a crucial role in temperature regulation. Ever wonder why you always feel cold when your thyroid is underactive? It's because low levels of thyroid hormones slow down your metabolic rate, making it harder for your body to generate heat. Conversely, an overactive thyroid can make you feel like you're in a perpetual sauna, as it revs up your metabolism and increases heat production.

The thyroid also has a hand in growth and development. In children, adequate thyroid hormone levels are critical for normal growth and brain development. For adults, these hormones are essential for maintaining healthy skin, hair, and nails. If you've noticed your hair thinning or your skin looking dry and flaky, your thyroid might be to blame.

Reproductive health is another area where the thyroid exerts its influence. Thyroid hormones interact with your sex hormones, affecting menstrual cycles and fertility. An underactive thyroid can lead to heavy, irregular periods, while an overactive thyroid can cause lighter, shorter cycles. This interaction doesn't stop at menstruation; thyroid imbalances can also affect your ability to conceive and maintain a pregnancy.

Like an old-fashioned thermostat, the body maintains thyroid hormone levels through intricate feedback loops. The hypothalamic-pituitary-thyroid (HPT) axis is the key player here. When your thyroid hormone levels drop, the hypothalamus releases thyrotropin-releasing hormone (TRH), which then prompts the pituitary gland to release TSH. This TSH stimulates the thyroid to produce more T3 and T4. Once levels are back to normal, the hypothalamus and pituitary get the signal to stop producing TRH and TSH. It's a delicate balancing act that keeps everything in check.

When this symbiotic relationship goes awry, the symptoms can be quite telling. Hyperthyroidism, or an overactive thyroid, can make you feel like you've had way too much caffeine. Symptoms include anxiety, palpitations, and an insatiable appetite. You might notice your heart racing even when you're just sitting down or feel jittery and anxious for no apparent reason.

On the flip side, hypothyroidism, or an underactive thyroid, can make you feel like you're moving through molasses. Fatigue, weight gain, and depression are common symptoms. You might struggle to get out of bed in the morning, feel sluggish throughout the day, and notice the numbers on the scale creeping up despite your best efforts.

Understanding how your thyroid interacts with other glands and influences various bodily functions can help you recognize when something is off. It's like being a savvy city planner; you don't need to know every detail, but understanding the big picture can make a world of difference. So, as we move forward, keep these relation-ships in mind. They're the key to unlocking the secrets of your thyroid health and ensuring that your tiny queen reigns supremely.

UNMASKING THE INVISIBLE TRIGGERS: ENVIRONMENTAL TOXINS AND VIRAL INFECTIONS

Let's talk about something that often flies under the radar but can have a significant impact on your thyroid—the invisible enemies lurking in your environment. Yes, I'm talking about environmental toxins and viral infections. You might not see them, but they're there, quietly messing with your thyroid function. Let's start with the usual suspects: heavy metals, pesticides, industrial pollutants, and sneaky endocrine-disrupting chemicals (EDCs) like BPA and phthalates.

Heavy metals, such as mercury and lead, are real troublemakers. They can sneak into your body through contaminated food, water, and air. Not to mention, silver fillings used by dentists a few decades ago and still today release toxic fumes in your mouth every time you eat or drink something hot. These metals can interfere with the production and regulation of thyroid hormones. They can cause oxidative stress, a condition where there's an imbalance between free radicals and antioxidants in your body.

This stress can damage your thyroid cells and lead to inflammation, making it harder for your thyroid to function properly. I had ten silver fillings from cavities when I was a kid. Just imagine how much heavy metal toxicity was built up in my body.

In case you're curious, here's some bonus information.

When searching for a local dentist who would safely remove my silver fillings, I stumbled across the International Academy of Oral Medicine and Toxicology website. I found a dentist who was SMART Certified by the IAOMT board. They even have a short video showing their process to keep you and the staff safe from mercury vapors during the removal process. I highly recommend checking to see if there is a dentist in your area or nearby if you have silver fillings and want to get them removed by visiting the International Academy of Oral Medicine and Toxicology website and do a search there for a SMART certified Dentist in your area.

The link to their website is-IAOMT Dentist Directory. You can also scan the QR code below.

Dietary strategies for detoxification are equally important. Incorporate detoxifying foods, such as leafy greens, cruciferous vegetables like broccoli and cauliflower, and citrus fruits into your diet. These foods are rich in antioxidants and nutrients that support your body's natural detox processes. Hydration is key, so ensure you drink plenty of water throughout the day. Water helps flush out toxins and keeps your body functioning smoothly. Herbal teas and detox smoothies can be a delicious way to support detoxification. Teas like dandelion root and nettle are known for their detoxifying properties, while smoothies packed with greens, fruits, and superfoods can give your liver a boost.

Maintaining a low-toxin lifestyle involves some ongoing habits. Regular physical activity is one of the best ways to promote detox-ification through sweating. Whether it's a brisk walk, a yoga session, or a workout at the gym, getting your sweat on helps elim-inate toxins through your skin. Saunas are another excellent option if you have access to one. Practicing intermittent fasting or detox diets periodically can also help. These practices give your digestive system a break and allow your body to focus on detoxifi-cation. Prioritizing organic and pesticide-free foods is another important step. Organic foods are grown without synthetic pesti-cides and herbicides, reducing your exposure to these harmful chemicals.

Making these changes doesn't have to be overwhelming. Start small and gradually incorporate more detox-friendly habits into your routine. You'll be amazed at how much better you feel when you reduce your body's toxic burden. Your thyroid will thank you, and you'll be on your way to a healthier, more vibrant life.

Now, let's move on to pesticides and herbicides. These chemicals are designed to kill pests but can also wreak havoc on your thyroid. You might be ingesting trace amounts of these chemicals when you consume non-organic fruits and vegetables. Over time, they can accumulate in your body and disrupt thyroid function. They can interfere with hormone production and exacerbate inflammation, making it even harder for your thyroid to do its job.

Industrial pollutants are another source of thyroid-disrupting toxins. These pollutants can be found in the air we breathe, the water we drink, and even the food we eat. Think of factories spewing out chemicals, cars emitting exhaust fumes, and pesticides sprayed on crops. Pesticides and herbicides, used to protect crops from pests and weeds, can also impact your thyroid. You might be ingesting trace amounts of these chemicals when you consume non-organic fruits and vegetables. Over time, they can accumulate in your body and disrupt your thyroid function.

Endocrine-disrupting chemicals (EDCs) are the silent saboteurs in this story. These are chemicals found in everyday products like plastics, cosmetics, and even canned foods. BPA (found in plastics) and phthalates (found in cosmetics) can mimic or interfere with your body's hormones, including thyroid hormones. Imagine them as pranksters who sneak into the castle and impersonate the queen's advisors, giving all the wrong orders. The result? Your thyroid gets confused, leading to imbalances that can manifest as fatigue, weight gain, or anxiety.

Picture this: you're cleaning your kitchen with your favorite lemon-scented cleaner, feeling all domestic goddess-like. You've got the windows open, and the sun is shining. But lurking in that fresh, citrusy scent might be chemicals that could mess with your thyroid. Household cleaners are one of the common sources of environmental toxins that can affect your thyroid health. Many of these products contain endocrine-disrupting chemicals (EDCs), which can interfere with hormone functions. Personal care products, like shampoos, lotions, and cosmetics, are also culprits. They often contain parabens and phthalates, which can sneak into your body through your skin.

So, how do these toxins wreak havoc on your thyroid? They mimic or interfere with your body's hormones, including thyroid hormones. Imagine them as unwelcome party crashers who mess up the music and disrupt the flow.

Reducing your exposure to these toxins is crucial for maintaining thyroid health. Start by choosing non-toxic household products. Look for cleaners that are free from harsh chemicals and opt for natural alternatives like vinegar and baking soda. When it comes to personal care, switch to products that are free from parabens, phthalates, and other harmful chemicals. Eating organic produce can also make a significant difference. Organic fruits and vegetables are grown without synthetic pesticides and herbicides, reducing your exposure to these toxins. Also, avoid using plastic containers, especially for storing or heating food. Many plastics contain BPA, an endocrine disruptor that can leach into your food and mess with your hormones.

Supporting your body's natural detoxification processes can further help mitigate the effects of these toxins. Your liver is your body's detox powerhouse, so supporting liver health is crucial. Milk thistle and dandelion root are herbs known for their liver-supporting properties. They help enhance liver function and promote the elimination of toxins. Consider incorporating these herbs into your routine through supplements or herbal teas. Detox diets and fasting can also be beneficial. These diets focus on consuming nutrient-dense foods that support detoxification, like leafy greens, cruciferous vegetables, and antioxidant-rich fruits.

Hydration is another key player in detoxification. Drinking plenty of water helps flush out toxins from your body. Aim for at least eight glasses a day, and consider adding a slice of lemon for an extra detox boost. Sweating is another effective way to eliminate toxins. Regular exercise, whether it's a brisk walk, a yoga session, or a gym workout, can help you work up a sweat and promote detoxification. Saunas are also great for sweating out toxins. If you have access to a sauna, consider incorporating regular sauna sessions into your routine.

By reducing exposure to environmental toxins and supporting your body's natural detox processes, you can help protect your thyroid health. It might feel overwhelming at first, but small changes can make a big difference. So, next time you're cleaning your kitchen or choosing a moisturizer, think about giving your thyroid the royal treatment it deserves.

Below is an example of some common endocrine-disrupting chemicals.

Common EDCs	Used In
Bisphenol A (BPA), Phthalates, Phenol	Plastics and Food Storage Materials
Brominated Flame Retardants, PCBs	Electronics and Building Materials
Phthalates, Parabens, UV Filters	Personal Care Products, Medical Tubing, sunscreen
Triclosan	Anti-Bacterial Soaps, Colgate Total

In case you're curious, here's some bonus information.

To learn more about EDCs, visit the Endocrine Society website at the link below or scan the QR code.

https://www.endocrine.org/patient-engagement/endocrine-library/edcs

But it's not just toxins we need to worry about. Viral infections can also play a significant role in triggering thyroid disorders. Take the Epstein-Barr virus (EBV), for instance. This virus, which causes mononucleosis (often called the kissing disease), can linger in your body long after the initial infection has passed. Studies suggest that EBV can trigger autoimmune thyroid diseases like Hashimoto's thyroiditis. It's as if the virus plants a seed of chaos that later blooms into full-blown thyroid dysfunction.

Hepatitis C is another viral culprit. This virus, primarily affecting the liver, has also been linked to thyroid issues. It's like having a double agent within your ranks, causing trouble in the liver and then sneaking over to disrupt your thyroid. Both EBV and Hepatitis C can trigger autoimmune responses, where your immune system starts attacking your own thyroid cells, mistaking them for invaders.

So, how exactly do these toxins and infections cause damage? The primary mechanisms are oxidative stress, inflammation, and autoimmune activation. Oxidative stress occurs when there's an imbalance between free radicals and antioxidants in your body. Free radicals are like little anarchists, causing cellular damage wherever they go. Inflammation is your body's natural response to injury or infection, but chronic inflammation can lead to tissue damage and autoimmune activation. When your immune system is constantly on high alert, it can start attacking your thyroid, mistaking it for an enemy.

Now that we've unmasked these invisible triggers let's talk about what you can do to protect yourself. First, consider detoxification strategies. This doesn't mean going on a juice cleanse for a week. Instead, focus on supporting your body's natural detox pathways. Drink plenty of water to flush out toxins, and incorporate foods rich in antioxidants, like berries, nuts, and green leafy vegetables, to combat oxidative stress.

Dietary recommendations are also crucial. Opt for organic produce whenever possible to reduce your exposure to pesticides and herbicides. Include seaweed and fish in your diet for iodine, but make sure they're from clean sources to avoid heavy metals. You might also want to consider supplements like selenium and zinc, which support thyroid function and help detoxify heavy metals.

Lifestyle changes can also make a big difference. Reduce your use of plastic containers and opt for glass or stainless steel instead. Avoid heating food in plastic, as this can cause chemicals like BPA to leach into your food. Choose natural, phthalate-free personal care products. And, of course, managing stress is essential. Chronic stress can exacerbate the effects of toxins and infections, so consider incorporating relaxation techniques like yoga or meditation into your daily routine.

In short, while you can't eliminate all environmental toxins or avoid viral infections entirely, you can take steps to minimize your exposure and support your body's ability to cope. By making informed choices about what you eat, how you live, and how you manage stress, you can help keep your thyroid—the tiny queen of your health—functioning at her best.

2

HER ROYAL STRUGGLE: THE THYROID QUEEN'S ROOT CAUSES AND RISK FACTORS

Picture this: you're sitting around the dinner table at a family reunion, and Aunt Linda starts talking about her thyroid issues. Before you know it, cousin Sally chimes in with her own thyroid saga, and then Grandma shares how she's been on medication since her 30s. You're starting to see a pattern here, aren't you? Well, you're not alone. Thyroid issues can often run in families, making them the not-so-fun family heirloom nobody asked for.

GENETIC PREDISPOSITIONS: THE FAMILY HEIRLOOM

Genetic factors play a significant role in thyroid disorders. If you have a family history of thyroid issues, your chances of experiencing similar problems increase. Think of it as inheriting your grandmother's antique necklace but with a less glamorous twist. Specific genes can predispose individuals to thyroid dysfunction. Research has shown that certain gene variants can increase the likelihood of developing autoimmune thyroid conditions like Hashimoto's thyroiditis and Graves' disease. It's like inheriting the family recipe for thyroid troubles, whether you want it or not.

Hashimoto's thyroiditis and Graves' disease are two of the most common inherited thyroid conditions. Hashimoto's thyroiditis, the leading cause of hypothyroidism in the United States, is an autoimmune disorder where your immune system mistakenly attacks your thyroid gland. It's like your body's defense system goes rogue, and instead of protecting you, it turns on you. Graves' disease, on the other hand, is an autoimmune disorder that causes hyperthyroidism. Your immune system produces antibodies that stimulate your thyroid to produce too much hormone, leading to a whirlwind of symptoms like rapid heartbeat, weight loss, and anxiety. Both conditions are like unwelcome relatives that crash every family gathering, causing chaos and disruption.

So, how do you know if you're genetically predisposed to thyroid issues? Genetic testing can provide valuable insights. It's like having a crystal ball that reveals your genetic blueprint. Genetic testing involves analyzing your DNA to identify specific gene variants associated with thyroid disorders. The benefits of genetic testing are numerous. It can help you understand your risk factors, allow for early detection, and enable proactive management of your thyroid health. To get tested, you can visit a healthcare provider specializing in genetic testing or use one of the many at-home genetic testing kits available online. Interpreting genetic test results can be tricky, so it's essential to consult with a healthcare professional who can help you understand what the results mean for you.

Managing genetic risk involves a combination of lifestyle modifications, regular screening, and early intervention strategies. First and foremost, adopting a healthy lifestyle can go a long way in supporting your thyroid health. A balanced diet rich in essential nutrients, regular exercise, and stress management techniques can help keep your thyroid in check. Think of it as giving your thyroid the royal treatment it deserves. Regular screening and monitoring are crucial, especially if you have a family history of thyroid disorders. Routine blood tests can help detect any changes in thyroid function early on, allowing for timely intervention. It's like having a royal guard that keeps a close watch on your thyroid, ensuring it stays in tip-top shape.

Early intervention strategies can make a significant difference in managing thyroid disorders. If you have a genetic predisposition, it's essential to work closely with your healthcare provider to develop a personalized plan. This plan may include dietary changes, supplements, and medications to support thyroid function. Additionally, staying informed about the latest research and treatments can empower you to make educated decisions about your health.

To make this information more actionable, consider the following checklist for managing genetic risk:

Genetic Risk Management Checklist

1. Consult with a healthcare provider: Discuss your family history and consider genetic testing.
2. Adopt a thyroid-friendly diet: Incorporate foods rich in iodine, selenium, and zinc.
3. Stay active: Engage in regular physical activity to support overall health.
4. Manage stress: Practice mindfulness, meditation, or yoga to reduce stress levels.
5. Regular screening: Schedule routine blood tests to monitor thyroid function.

By following this checklist, you can take proactive steps to manage your genetic risk and support your thyroid health. Remember, while you can't change your genes, you have the power to influence how they affect your health through informed choices and proactive management. So, let's give your thyroid the royal treatment it deserves and keep it reigning supremely!

STRESS AND THE THYROID: A DELICATE BALANCE

Imagine you're running late for work, juggling your coffee, keys, and phone, when suddenly your boss calls with an urgent request. Your heart races, your palms get sweaty, and you feel like you're in panic mode. That's stress in action, and while it's normal in small doses, chronic stress can wreak havoc on your thyroid. When you're stressed, your body releases a hormone called cortisol. Think of cortisol as your body's built-in alarm system. It's great for short-term emergencies, like running from a saber-toothed tiger (or your child breaks their arm from falling out of a tree), but not so great when it's constantly elevated. High cortisol levels can inhibit the production of thyroid hormones, leading to a sluggish thyroid. Over time, this chronic stress can deplete your adrenal glands, resulting in adrenal fatigue, which further complicates thyroid function.

Chronic stress doesn't just mess with hormone production; it can also pave the way for thyroid disorders. When your body is in a constant state of stress, your immune system can go haywire. This is where autoimmune thyroid conditions like Hashimoto's thyroiditis and Graves' disease come into play. Chronic stress can trigger these conditions by causing your immune system to attack your thyroid gland, mistaking it for an invader. It's like your body's security system is going rogue and attacking the thing it's supposed to protect. Even if you already have a thyroid condition, chronic stress can worsen your symptoms, making it feel like you're stuck in an endless cycle of fatigue, anxiety, and weight gain.

So, how do you break this cycle? The answer lies in stress management techniques that can support your thyroid health. One powerful tool is mindfulness meditation. Practicing mindfulness can train your mind to stay in the present moment, reducing the constant chatter of worries and "what-ifs." Start with just a few minutes a day, focusing on your breath and letting go of any distracting thoughts. Another effective technique is yoga. This gentle form of exercise not only stretches and strengthens your body but also calms your mind. Try incorporating yoga into your routine a few times a week to help reduce stress and improve your overall well-being. Time management and setting boundaries are also crucial. Make a to-do list and prioritize tasks, allowing yourself to say no when your plate is already full. Remember, you can't pour from an empty cup.

Let's look at a real-life example. Meet Savannah, a high-powered executive who was always on the go. She thrived on deadlines and loved her fast-paced job, but the constant stress took a toll on her health over time. She started experiencing extreme fatigue, weight gain, and mood swings. After months of struggling, she was diagnosed with stress-induced hypothyroidism. Determined to take control of her health, Savannah decided to make some changes. She started practicing mindfulness meditation every morning, joined a local yoga class, and set strict boundaries between her work and personal life. Over time, she noticed a significant improvement in her symptoms. Her energy levels increased, she began to lose weight, and her mood stabilized. Savannah's journey is a testament to the power of stress management in supporting thyroid health.

Savannah's story isn't unique. Many women in perimenopause experience similar challenges. The hormonal fluctuations of perimenopause can amplify the effects of stress, making it even more essential to find effective stress management techniques. For example, Lisa is a mother of two and a small business owner. Lisa was always juggling multiple responsibilities, leaving little time for herself. She began experiencing symptoms like fatigue, irritability, and weight gain. After a visit to her doctor, she learned that her stress levels were exacerbating her thyroid condition. Lisa decided to make some changes. She started by setting aside time each day for self-care, whether it was a walk in the park, a hot bath, or simply reading a book. She also began practicing yoga and found it to be incredibly beneficial in reducing her stress levels. With these changes, Lisa significantly improved her symptoms and felt more in control of her health.

Incorporating stress management techniques into your routine doesn't have to be complicated. Start small and find what works best for you. Whether it's mindfulness meditation, yoga, or simply taking time for yourself, these practices can make a big difference in supporting your thyroid health. Remember, managing stress isn't just about reducing anxiety; it's about giving your thyroid the royal treatment it deserves. So, take a deep breath, roll out that yoga mat, and know that you're taking steps towards a healthier, happier you.

AUTOIMMUNE RESPONSES: WHEN THE BODY TURNS AGAINST ITSELF

Imagine your immune system as a diligent security team, always looking for intruders like bacteria and viruses. But what happens when this team gets confused and starts attacking your own body? This is the essence of autoimmune diseases. In the case of thyroid health, it's like your immune system has mistaken your thyroid gland for an invader and launched a full-scale attack. This malfunction leads to the production of autoantibodies, which are like misguided missiles targeting your thyroid cells. These autoantibodies can damage the thyroid, disrupting its ability to produce hormones effectively.

Two common autoimmune thyroid conditions are Hashimoto's thyroiditis and Graves' disease. Hashimoto's thyroiditis is the more prevalent of the two and primarily results in hypothyroidism. Symptoms can include fatigue, weight gain, and depression, among others. It's diagnosed through blood tests that reveal elevated levels of thyroid peroxidase (TPO) antibodies, which indicate that your immune system is attacking your thyroid. On the other hand, Graves' disease leads to hyperthyroidism. Symptoms for Graves' include anxiety, rapid heartbeat, and unexplained weight loss. Diagnosis often involves blood tests showing low TSH levels and high levels of thyroid-stimulating immunoglobulins (TSIs), which essentially trick your thyroid into overproducing hormones.

Various triggers can set off these autoimmune responses. Infections and viruses are one such trigger. Imagine catching a common cold and, somewhere along the line, your immune system gets its wires crossed, leading to an autoimmune attack on your thyroid. Dietary triggers can also play a role. For some people, consuming gluten or dairy can exacerbate autoimmune thyroid conditions. It's like your favorite comfort foods turning into hidden enemies. Emotional stress and trauma can also be significant triggers, as stress hormones can wreak havoc on your immune system, making it more likely to attack your thyroid.

Managing autoimmune thyroid conditions often requires a multifaceted approach. One effective strategy is adopting an anti-inflammatory diet, such as the Autoimmune Protocol (AIP). This diet focuses on eliminating foods that can trigger inflammation and autoimmune responses, like gluten, dairy, and processed foods while emphasizing nutrient-dense foods like vegetables, fruits, and lean proteins. It's like giving your thyroid a much-needed vacation from irritants. Supplements can also support immune health. Selenium, for example, has been shown to reduce thyroid antibodies, while omega-3 fatty acids can help reduce inflammation.

Medical treatments are often necessary to manage these conditions effectively. For those with Hashimoto's, thyroid hormone replacement therapy can help normalize hormone levels, alleviating symptoms like fatigue and weight gain. It's akin to giving your thyroid a little help to keep the kingdom running smoothly. In cases of Graves' disease, treatments may include antithyroid medications that reduce hormone production or, in more severe cases, radioactive iodine therapy to shrink the thyroid gland. Immunosuppressants might also be prescribed to help calm the immune system's overactive response.

To make these management strategies more actionable, consider incorporating the following elements into your daily routine:

Autoimmune Thyroid Management Checklist

1. Follow an Anti-Inflammatory Diet: Adopt the AIP diet to reduce inflammation and support thyroid health.
2. Take Supportive Supplements: Incorporate selenium, omega-3 fatty acids, and other immune-supporting supplements into your regimen.
3. Monitor Symptoms and Hormone Levels: Regularly check your thyroid hormone levels and adjust treatments as needed.

4. Manage Stress: Practice stress-reducing activities like mindfulness meditation, yoga, or spending time in nature.
5. Consult with a Functional Medicine Doctor or an Integrative Doctor: Work closely with your doctor to develop and adjust your treatment plan.

Understanding the autoimmune nature of these thyroid conditions and adopting a comprehensive management plan can help you take control of your health. While it might sometimes feel overwhelming, remember that with the right strategies and support, you can navigate these challenges and support your thyroid's royal reign.

THE ROLE OF HORMONAL CHANGES: THYROID HEALTH DURING PERIMENOPAUSE

Perimenopause is like a hormonal roller coaster that no one asked to ride. One minute you're fine, the next you're dealing with hot flashes, mood swings, and a body that seems to have a mind of its own. During this phase, there's a significant decline in estrogen and progesterone levels. This hormonal shift can throw your thyroid for a loop, as these hormones play a crucial role in maintaining thyroid function. When estrogen levels drop, it can affect thyroid-binding globulin (TBG), a protein that transports thyroid hormones in your bloodstream. Lower estrogen means less TBG, resulting in more free thyroid hormones floating around. This can disrupt the delicate balance your thyroid strives to maintain.

The symptoms of thyroid dysfunction and perimenopause often overlap, making it tricky to pinpoint the root cause of your discomfort. Fatigue is a common complaint. You might feel drained, even after a full night's sleep. Mood swings are another shared symptom. One moment, you're calm, and the next, you're snapping at your loved ones for no apparent reason. Weight gain is a double whammy during this time. Your slowing metabolism, courtesy of both thyroid issues and hormonal changes, makes it more challenging to shed those extra pounds. And let's not forget hot flashes, which can leave you feeling like you're living in a sauna. Sleep disturbances and cognitive issues, such as brain fog and memory lapses, add to the frustration. It's like your body is conspiring against you, leaving you to wonder if you'll ever feel normal again.

So, what can you do to manage these hormonal changes and support your thyroid? One option is hormone replacement therapy (HRT). HRT involves taking medications that contain female hormones to replace the ones your body no longer makes. This can help alleviate some of the symptoms of perimenopause and support thyroid function. However, HRT isn't suitable for everyone, so it's essential to discuss the risks and benefits with your healthcare provider. For those seeking natural alternatives, phytoestrogens and other natural supplements can be a viable option. Phytoestrogens are plant-based compounds that mimic estrogen in the body. Foods like soy, flaxseeds, lentils, apples, and pinto beans are rich in phytoestrogens and can help balance hormone levels. You can also google to get a longer list of foods that are phytoestrogen-rich.

Lifestyle modifications are another crucial aspect of managing hormonal changes. A balanced diet that supports thyroid health is vital. Focus on nutrient-dense foods rich in iodine, selenium, and zinc. These nutrients play a significant role in thyroid function. Regular exercise can also make a world of difference. Not only does it help manage weight, but it also boosts mood and energy levels. Aim for a mix of cardio, strength training, and flexibility exercises to keep your body in top shape. Stress management is equally important. Techniques like yoga, mindfulness meditation, and deep breathing exercises can help reduce stress levels and support thyroid health.

Let's turn to some real-life stories to see how others have navigated this challenging phase. Meet Emma, a 45-year-old teacher who started experiencing perimenopausal symptoms along with hypothyroidism. She found herself constantly tired, gaining weight, and dealing with mood swings that affected her work and personal life. After discussing her options with her doctor, Emma decided to try HRT. Within a few months, she noticed a significant improvement in her energy levels and mood. She also made dietary changes, incorporating more phytoestrogen-rich foods and taking selenium supplements. Emma's experience highlights the importance of a personalized approach to managing hormonal changes.

Another inspiring story comes from Jane, who shared her journey in a support group. Jane struggled with hot flashes, insomnia, and brain fog, all while managing her thyroid condition. She opted for natural supplements and lifestyle changes instead of HRT. Jane started practicing yoga and mindfulness meditation, which helped her manage stress and improve her sleep. She also made dietary adjustments, focusing on whole foods and avoiding processed sugars. Over time, Jane found that these changes significantly enhanced her symptoms, allowing her to feel more in control of her health.

These stories underline the importance of finding what works best for you. Whether it's HRT, natural supplements, lifestyle modifications, or a combination, the goal is to support your thyroid and manage the hormonal fluctuations of perimenopause. Remember, it's all about giving your body the care and attention it deserves during this transformative phase. Taking proactive steps can help you navigate perimenopause with confidence and maintain your thyroid health.

As we've explored, perimenopause can significantly impact thyroid health, but with the right strategies, you can manage these changes effectively. In the next chapter, we'll dive into the symptoms and diagnosis of thyroid disorders, helping you understand the signs to watch for and how to get a proper diagnosis. Your thyroid journey continues here, with more insights and practical tips to keep you feeling your best.

3

THE QUEEN'S DILEMMA: DECODING DISORDERS THAT DISTURB HER RULE

Imagine waking up one day and feeling like you're walking through molasses. Every step is an effort, every task feels monumental, and no amount of coffee seems to lift the fog. This is the reality for many women with hypothyroidism, a condition where your thyroid gland fails to produce enough hormones to keep your body running smoothly. Let's dive into the nitty-gritty of what happens when your thyroid decides to go on strike and how you can reclaim your energy and vitality.

HYPOTHYROIDISM: THE UNDERACTIVE THYROID

Welcome to the world of hypothyroidism, where your thyroid has decided to take a prolonged nap. Hypothyroidism is when your thyroid gland doesn't produce enough thyroid hormones. The most common culprit? Hashimoto's thyroiditis is an autoimmune condition where your immune system mistakenly attacks your thyroid. Another cause is iodine deficiency, which can throw a wrench into the works because iodine is crucial for thyroid hormone production. Without enough iodine, your thyroid can't churn out the hormones your body needs, leaving you feeling slug-gish and out of sorts.

Hypothyroidism occurs when your thyroid gland doesn't produce enough thyroid hormones. Think of it as the queen being too tired to run the kingdom. There are two main types: primary hypothy-roidism and secondary hypothyroidism. In primary hypothy-roidism, the problem lies within the thyroid gland itself. It's like the queen has locked herself in her room and refuses to come out. This can happen due to autoimmune disorders like Hashimoto's thyroiditis, where your immune system mistakenly attacks your thyroid. Iodine deficiency can also cause primary hypothyroidism because iodine is crucial for thyroid hormone production. Previous thyroid surgery or radiation treatment can leave your thyroid unable to produce enough hormones.

Secondary hypothyroidism, on the other hand, is a bit more complex. Here, the issue originates from the pituitary gland, which is supposed to signal the thyroid to produce hormones. It's like the queen's advisor (the pituitary gland) is giving the wrong orders or no orders at all. This can happen due to pituitary tumors, surgery, radiation, or the disruption of normal hormone production from the build-up of heavy metals.

The symptoms of hypothyroidism can sneak up on you and are often mistaken for just "getting older" or "being tired." Chronic fatigue and sluggishness are the most common complaints. You might feel like no amount of sleep is ever enough, and dragging yourself out of bed in the morning feels like a Herculean task. Weight gain despite normal diet and exercise is another telltale sign. It's frustrating to watch the scale climb when you're doing everything right. Cold intolerance is also common; you might be shivering while everyone else is comfortable or constantly reaching for an extra blanket.

Other symptoms can include dry skin, hair loss, and muscle weakness. Your skin might feel like sandpaper, and your hair could start thinning or falling out more than usual. Muscle weakness can make simple tasks feel exhausting, and you might notice a general slowing down in your movements and speech. It's as if your entire body is operating on low power mode.

So, why does hypothyroidism develop? Autoimmune disorders like Hashimoto's thyroiditis are the most common cause in iodine-sufficient areas. In Hashimoto's, your immune system creates antibodies that attack your thyroid, gradually destroying its ability to produce hormones. Iodine deficiency, while less common in developed countries, can still be a cause if your diet is lacking in iodine. Previous thyroid surgery or radiation treatment can also leave your thyroid unable to produce enough hormones, leading to hypothyroidism.

Diagnosing hypothyroidism involves a few key steps. Blood tests are the frontline tool. Your doctor should check your levels of TSH (thyroid-stimulating hormone), free T4 (thyroxine), free T3 (triiodothyronine), reverse T3, TPO (thyroid peroxidase), and TG (Thyroglobulin). TPO (thyroid peroxidase) and TG (Thyroglobulin) are thyroid antibodies. Thyroid antibodies form when the immune system mistakenly targets the thyroid's cells and tissues. This can result in inflammation, tissue damage, or impaired thyroid function. These antibodies are responsible for autoimmune thyroid conditions like Graves' disease and Hashimoto's thyroiditis.

Elevated TSH and low Free T4 levels indicate hypothyroidism. It's like the pituitary gland is shouting at the thyroid to produce more hormones, but the thyroid isn't responding. Once diagnosed, the mainstay treatment is levothyroxine therapy, a synthetic form of the T4 hormone. This medication helps restore normal hormone levels, alleviate symptoms, and allow you to feel more like yourself again. In my case, I was prescribed levothyroxine. It seemed to help a little bit, but after six months of being on levothyroxine, my doctor said my T3 was still too low and wanted to switch me to a different thyroid medication. She explained that sometimes our bodies can't always convert the synthetic T4 into T3. This is why monitoring your thyroid levels and making adjustments, if necessary, is vital. I later learned that only a small population does well on the T4 prescription.

Regular monitoring and dosage adjustments are crucial in managing hypothyroidism. Your doctor will likely recommend periodic blood tests to ensure your hormone levels are stable. This proactive approach can make you feel empowered and in control of your health, much like fine-tuning a musical instrument; sometimes, it takes a few tweaks to get everything in harmony.

To help you stay on track, here's a simple checklist:

Hypothyroidism Management Checklist

1. Regular Blood Tests: Schedule blood tests every 3-6 months to monitor all your thyroid hormones.
2. Diet: Incorporate iodine-rich foods like fish, dairy, and iodized salt.
3. Lifestyle: Engage in regular exercise and manage stress through relaxation techniques.

Understanding and managing hypothyroidism can feel overwhelming, but with the right knowledge and support, you can navigate this condition and reclaim your vitality and energy. With proper management, you can lead a fulfilling life full of energy and vitality despite the challenges of hypothyroidism.

HYPERTHYROIDISM: THE OVERACTIVE THYROID

Imagine feeling like you've had ten cups of coffee all at once, but you haven't touched a drop. Your heart races, you're sweating buckets, and you can't seem to sit still. Welcome to the world of hyperthyroidism, where your thyroid gland is working overtime. This condition occurs when the thyroid produces excessive amounts of T3 (triiodothyronine) and T4 (thyroxine) hormones, cranking up your metabolic rate to warp speed. It's like the queen has decided to throw a never-ending festival, and everyone in the kingdom is running around in high gear.

The symptoms of hyperthyroidism can be both startling and debilitating. One of the most noticeable signs is a rapid heartbeat, often accompanied by palpitations. You might feel like your heart is trying to leap out of your chest, even when you're just sitting quietly. Unintended weight loss is another common symptom. Despite eating normally or even more than usual, you might find the pounds melting away. This might sound like a dream come true for some, but it's usually a sign that something's off. Nervousness and irritability can also plague you, making it hard to relax or enjoy your day. Heat intolerance and excessive sweating are other frustrating symptoms. You might feel unbearably hot all the time, even when everyone else is comfortable, and find yourself sweating profusely with minimal exertion.

So, what causes this thyroid overdrive? The most common culprit is Graves' disease, an autoimmune disorder where your immune system produces antibodies that stimulate the thyroid to produce too much hormone. It's like the queen's advisors are giving her a never-ending list of tasks, and she's frantically trying to keep up. Toxic adenomas, which are lumps in the thyroid that produce excess hormones, can also lead to hyperthyroidism. Thyroiditis, or inflammation of the thyroid, can cause a temporary spike in hormone levels as the gland releases stored hormones into the bloodstream.

Diagnosing hyperthyroidism involves several steps. Blood tests are the first line of defense, checking levels of TSH, Free T3, and Free T4. In hyperthyroidism, TSH levels are usually low because the pituitary gland tries to slow down hormone production, while Free T3 and Free T4 levels are elevated. A radioactive iodine uptake test can provide more information. This test measures how much iodine your thyroid absorbs, which helps identify the cause of hyperthyroidism.

Treatment options vary based on the severity and cause of the condition. Antithyroid medications like Methimazole can help reduce hormone production. These medications act like a brake, slowing down the overactive thyroid. Beta-blockers are often prescribed to manage symptoms like rapid heartbeat and palpitations. They don't address the underlying cause but can help you feel more comfortable. For more severe cases, radioactive iodine therapy is a common treatment. This involves taking a radioactive iodine pill that selectively destroys overactive thyroid cells, reducing hormone production. Surgery, or thyroidectomy, is another option, especially if other treatments aren't effective or if there's a large goiter.

Managing hyperthyroidism can be challenging, but understanding the condition and working closely with your healthcare provider can help you regain control. Regular monitoring and follow-up appointments are crucial to ensure your treatment is effective and to adjust dosages as needed. It's like keeping a close eye on the kingdom to ensure everything runs smoothly. Navigating hyperthyroidism involves knowing the signs, understanding the causes, and exploring the various treatment options available. With the right approach, you can manage this condition and live a balanced, healthy life.

HASHIMOTO'S DISEASE: THE AUTOIMMUNE ATTACK

Imagine your immune system as a vigilant guard dog, always on the lookout for intruders. In the case of Hashimoto's disease, this guard dog goes rogue, attacking the very thing it's supposed to protect: your thyroid gland. Hashimoto's, also known as chronic lymphocytic thyroiditis, is an autoimmune disorder where your immune system creates antibodies against thyroid peroxidase (TPO) and thyroglobulin. These antibodies are like misguided missiles, targeting and gradually destroying your thyroid cells. This autoimmune assault leads to chronic inflammation and fibrosis, slowly disabling your thyroid's ability to produce hormones effectively.

Hashimoto's often sneaks up on you, with symptoms that develop gradually over time. Unlike other thyroid disorders, Hashimoto's is a slow burn. You may start with mild symptoms like fatigue and muscle weakness, which can easily be mistaken for just being overworked. But as the condition progresses, you might notice more pronounced signs like the formation of a goiter or an enlarged thyroid gland that can make swallowing or even breathing a chore. Fatigue becomes a constant companion, and muscle weakness can make everyday tasks feel like climbing Mount Everest. This slow onset can make Hashimoto's tricky to diagnose early, often leaving you feeling frustrated and misunderstood.

So, what makes someone more likely to develop Hashimoto's? Genetic predisposition plays a significant role. If you have a family history of autoimmune diseases, you're more likely to develop Hashimoto's. Environmental triggers, such as stress and infections, can also set off the autoimmune response. It's like throwing gasoline on a smoldering fire. Women are more prone to Hashimoto's, with the condition being ten times more common in women than men. Hormonal changes, particularly during pregnancy, menopause, or periods of high stress, can act as triggers. It's like your thyroid is extra sensitive to the hormonal roller coasters that women often face.

Diagnosing Hashimoto's involves a combination of blood tests and imaging. Blood tests for TPO antibodies are a key diagnostic tool. Elevated levels of these antibodies indicate that your immune system is attacking your thyroid. A thyroid ultrasound can provide a closer look at the gland, revealing characteristic changes like an enlarged, lumpy thyroid with areas of fibrosis. Once diagnosed, the primary treatment is levothyroxine or a natural thyroid hormone tablet, and the two big-name brands are NP Thyroid and Armour Thyroid.

However, addressing the underlying autoimmune activity is equally important. Managing stress through mindfulness, yoga, or other relaxation techniques can help reduce the autoimmune response. A diet rich in anti-inflammatory foods, like leafy greens, berries, and fatty fish, can also support your thyroid. Avoiding gluten and dairy might benefit some, as these foods can exacerbate autoimmune symptoms. Regular monitoring and follow-up appointments with your healthcare provider are essential. Adjusting medication dosages based on your hormone levels and symptoms ensures that you're getting the right amount of support.

To help you navigate Hashimoto's, consider incorporating a few practical steps into your routine. Start by paying attention to your body's signals, and don't ignore persistent symptoms like fatigue or muscle weakness. Make dietary changes that focus on anti-inflammatory foods and consider eliminating potential triggers like gluten. Practice stress management techniques regularly to keep your immune system in check. Most importantly, work closely with your healthcare provider to monitor your condition and adjust treatments as needed.

Understanding Hashimoto's disease and its impact on your thyroid health can empower you to take control of your well-being. While it may feel overwhelming at times, remember that with the right strategies and support, you can manage this condition and live a balanced, healthy life.

GRAVES' DISEASE: WHEN THE IMMUNE SYSTEM OVERREACTS

Imagine your immune system as a hyperactive security guard who can't tell friend from foe. That's basically what happens in Graves' disease. This autoimmune disorder leads to hyperthyroidism by causing your immune system to produce thyroid-stimulating immunoglobulins (TSIs). These TSIs act like overly enthusiastic cheerleaders, constantly telling your thyroid to produce more hormones. The result? An overstimulated thyroid gland that's working overtime, cranking out excessive amounts of T3 and T4 hormones.

The symptoms of Graves' disease can be quite dramatic. One of the most unique and noticeable signs is exophthalmos or bulging eyes. It's not just a slight puffiness; we're talking about eyes that seem to be popping out of their sockets. This can also lead to double vision, making everyday tasks like reading or driving a real challenge. Another symptom is pretibial myxedema, which causes the skin on your shins to thicken and take on a lumpy, reddish appearance. It's like your body is throwing all sorts of weird symptoms your way, making it hard to ignore that something is seriously off.

So, what triggers this overzealous immune response? Genetic factors play a significant role. If you have a family history of Graves' disease or other autoimmune conditions, you're more likely to develop it. Stress and infections can also act as triggers, setting off an immune response that spirals out of control. Smoking is another risk factor. Not only does it increase the likelihood of developing Graves' disease, but it can also worsen the symptoms, especially the eye-related ones. It's like adding fuel to the fire, making an already bad situation worse.

Diagnosing Graves' disease involves a series of tests. Blood tests for TSIs can confirm the presence of these rogue antibodies. Elevated levels of TSIs are a clear sign that your immune system is overstimulating your thyroid. A radioactive iodine uptake test can also be helpful. In this test, you swallow a small amount of radioactive iodine, and your thyroid absorbs it. The amount of iodine your thyroid takes up can help diagnose the cause of your hyperthyroidism.

Treatment options for Graves' disease are varied and depend on the severity of your symptoms. Antithyroid medications can help reduce hormone production. These drugs act like a dampener, slowing down the overactive thyroid. Beta-blockers are often prescribed to manage symptoms like rapid heartbeat and palpitations. They don't address the underlying cause but can make you feel more comfortable. Radioactive iodine therapy is another common treatment. This involves taking a radioactive iodine pill that selectively destroys overactive thyroid cells, reducing hormone production. For more severe or persistent cases, surgical removal of the thyroid, or thyroidectomy, may be necessary. This option is usually considered when other treatments aren't effective or if there's a large goiter causing symptoms.

Managing Graves' disease can be challenging, but understanding the condition and working closely with your healthcare provider can help you regain control. Regular monitoring and follow-up appointments are crucial to ensure your treatment is effective and to adjust dosages as needed. Your immune system might be over-reacting, but with the right approach, you can manage this condition and live a balanced, healthy life. Throughout this process, it's essential to focus on both the physical and emotional aspects of your well-being. Remember, you're not alone in this, and there are multiple avenues to explore for effective management.

THYROID NODULES AND GOITER: WHAT YOU NEED TO KNOW

Imagine waking up one morning, looking in the mirror, and noticing a slight swelling in your neck. Panic sets in. What is that lump? Is it something serious? Welcome to the world of thyroid nodules and goiters. Thyroid nodules are lumps that form within the thyroid gland. They can be solitary or multiple and vary in size. Sometimes, they're so small you wouldn't even know they're there without an ultrasound. In contrast, a goiter is an enlarged thyroid gland. Think of it as your thyroid throwing a tantrum and deciding to make itself more noticeable.

These conditions can manifest in a variety of ways. The most obvious sign is visible swelling in the neck, which can sometimes be so pronounced that it looks like you're harboring a small tennis ball. This can lead to difficulty swallowing or breathing as the enlarged thyroid presses against the trachea and esophagus. While most nodules are benign, there's always a slight risk they could be cancerous. That's why any new lump should be evaluated by a healthcare provider. The mere thought of a nodule being cancerous is enough to send anyone into a spiral of worry.

So, what causes these thyroid hiccups? Iodine deficiency is a major culprit. Your thyroid needs iodine to produce hormones, and without enough iodine, it can become enlarged or develop nodules. Hashimoto's disease, where your immune system attacks your thyroid, can also lead to nodules and goiter. Genetic factors play a role, too. If thyroid issues run in your family, you might be more prone to developing them. Radiation exposure, whether from medical treatments or environmental factors, can increase the risk as well.

Diagnosing thyroid nodules and goiters involves a combination of physical examinations and imaging studies. During a physical exam, your doctor will feel your neck for any enlargements or lumps. An ultrasound is often the next step. This imaging test uses sound waves to create a picture of your thyroid, helping to determine the size and nature of any nodules. If a nodule looks suspicious, a fine-needle aspiration biopsy might be performed. This involves using a thin needle to extract cells from the nodule for further examination under a microscope. It sounds scarier than it is, and it's a crucial step in ruling out cancer.

Treatment options depend on the size, nature, and symptoms of the nodules or goiter. For small, benign nodules that aren't causing symptoms, regular monitoring might be all that's needed. This involves periodic ultrasounds to ensure they're not growing or changing. If a nodule is suspicious or causing symptoms, surgical intervention might be necessary. Removing part or all of the thyroid can eliminate the problem, though it may require lifelong thyroid hormone replacement therapy. For goiters, treatment focuses on addressing the underlying cause. If it's due to iodine deficiency, iodine supplements might be recommended. In cases where the goiter is large or causing symptoms, surgery might be the best option.

Living with thyroid nodules or goiters can be stressful, but understanding the condition and knowing what to expect can make it more manageable. Regular check-ups and open communication with your healthcare provider are key to staying on top of your thyroid health. While the idea of a lump in your neck can be unsettling, it's important to remember that most thyroid nodules are benign and treatable.

THYROID CANCER: EARLY DETECTION AND TREATMENT OPTIONS

You're sitting at your desk, minding your own business, when you feel a lump in your neck. Panic sets in. Could it be thyroid cancer? Let's break down what you need to know about the different types of thyroid cancer and how to catch it early. Thyroid cancer isn't as common as other thyroid disorders, but it's important to know what to look for and what to expect.

First, let's talk about the types of thyroid cancer. Papillary thyroid cancer is the most common type, accounting for about 80% of cases. It's slow-growing and often found in one lobe of the thyroid. Think of it as the tortoise of thyroid cancers—it moves slowly but steadily. Follicular thyroid cancer is the next most common type. It's also slow-growing but has a higher chance of spreading to other parts of the body, like the lungs or bones. Medullary thyroid cancer is less common and can be part of a genetic syndrome. It's like the black sheep of the thyroid cancer family, often running in families and requiring special attention. The rarest and most aggressive type is anaplastic thyroid cancer. It's fast-growing and difficult to treat, making it the hare in our cancer analogy.

So, how do you know if you should be worried about thyroid cancer? The most common symptom is a lump or nodule in the neck. This lump might be painless or cause some discomfort. Hoarseness or voice changes can also be a sign that something's not right, especially if these changes persist. Difficulty swallowing is another red flag. If you find it hard to get food down, or you feel like there's something stuck in your throat, it's time to see a doctor. These symptoms can be subtle, but they're worth paying attention to.

Now, let's discuss what could increase your risk of developing thyroid cancer. Family history is a significant factor. If thyroid cancer runs in your family, your risk is higher. Genetic syndromes, like multiple endocrine neoplasia (MEN), can also increase your risk. Radiation exposure, whether from medical treatments or environmental factors, is another risk factor. Women are more likely to develop thyroid cancer than men, and it's most common in adults, particularly those over 40. Understanding these risk factors can help you stay vigilant and proactive about your health.

Detecting thyroid cancer involves several steps. An ultrasound is usually the first test. It creates images of your thyroid, helping doctors see if there are any suspicious lumps or nodules. If anything looks concerning, a biopsy is the next step. This involves using a thin needle to extract cells from the nodule, which are then examined under a microscope. Blood tests for calcitonin and other cancer markers can also provide valuable information. These tests help confirm the diagnosis and determine the best course of treatment.

When it comes to treatment, surgical removal of the thyroid, or thyroidectomy, is often the first step. This surgery removes the thyroid gland, eliminating the primary source of cancer. Radioactive iodine treatment is another option. This treatment involves swallowing a radioactive iodine pill that targets and destroys any remaining cancer cells. For more advanced cases, targeted therapies and chemotherapy may be necessary. These treatments focus on destroying cancer cells while minimizing damage to healthy tissue. The goal is to eliminate the cancer and prevent it from coming back.

Living with thyroid cancer can be challenging, but early detection and effective treatment can make a significant difference. Regular check-ups and open communication with your healthcare provider are crucial. Stay informed about your condition and treatment options, and don't hesitate to ask questions or seek a second opinion if needed. Knowledge is power, and understanding your condition can help you make informed decisions about your health.

Diagnosing these thyroid disorders involves a mix of detective work and medical tests. Blood tests are the frontline tools, measuring levels of TSH, T3, and T4. High TSH and low T4 point towards hypothyroidism, while low TSH and high T4 suggest hyperthyroidism. Imaging studies, like ultrasounds, can provide a closer look at the thyroid's structure, revealing nodules or inflammation. Sometimes, a radioactive iodine uptake test is used to see how much iodine your thyroid absorbs, which can help pinpoint the exact nature of the issue.

The symptoms of thyroid disorders can be a mixed bag, making them tricky to pin down. For hypothyroidism, think fatigue, weight gain, and mood swings. You might feel like you're moving through a fog, with dry skin, thinning hair, and a constant chill as your unwelcome companions. On the flip side, hyperthyroidism can make you feel like you've had one too many espressos. Anxiety, palpitations, weight loss, and increased sweating are common signs. You might notice your eyes bulging slightly or feel like you're always running hot, no matter the weather.

Let's bring this to life with an everyday example. Imagine you're a busy mom, juggling work, kids, and a million other things. You've noticed you're more tired than usual, and despite eating a balanced diet, you're gaining weight. Your mood swings are starting to worry your family, and your hair seems to be falling out more than normal. After a visit to your doctor and some blood tests, you find out you have hypothyroidism, likely caused by Hashimoto's thyroiditis. The diagnosis might feel overwhelming, but it's also a relief to know there's a reason behind your symptoms.

Understanding these common thyroid disorders is the first step in taking control of your health. As we explore further in the book, we'll dive into natural remedies, lifestyle changes, and treatment options that can help manage these conditions. Whether you're dealing with a sluggish thyroid, an overactive one, or something in between, there's hope and help available. Your thyroid might be small, but with the right knowledge and support, you can navigate these challenges and reclaim your energy and well-being.

4

THE QUEEN'S TEST: DIAGNOSING
THYROID ISSUES IN HER ROYAL
DOMAIN

Imagine this: you're sitting in the doctor's office, waiting for your blood test results. Your mind is racing. Did I remember to take my meds this morning? Is my coffee addiction finally catching up with me? The doctor walks in with a serious look, and you brace yourself. "We need to talk about your thyroid blood panel," he says. Suddenly, it feels like you're back in high school, waiting for grades on a test you didn't study for. But don't worry; I'm here to help you decode this mysterious panel of numbers and letters.

UNDERSTANDING THYROID BLOOD PANELS: READING BETWEEN THE LINES

Let's start with the basics. Your thyroid blood panel is like a report card for your thyroid gland. It tells you how well your thyroid is functioning and can help diagnose issues like hypothyroidism or hyperthyroidism. The key components of this panel are Thyroid Stimulating Hormone (TSH), Free T4 (Thyroxine), Free T3 (Triiodothyronine), and Reverse T3. Each of these measurements provides a piece of the puzzle.

TSH is produced by your pituitary gland and acts like a manager, telling your thyroid how much hormone to produce. Think of TSH as the queen's advisor, whispering orders to keep the kingdom running smoothly. When TSH levels are high, it means your thyroid isn't producing enough hormones, and your pituitary gland is working overtime to compensate. This is a common indicator of hypothyroidism. On the flip side, low TSH levels suggest that your thyroid is overactive and producing too much hormone, a sign of hyperthyroidism.

Next up, we have Free T4, the inactive form of thyroid hormone. Free T4 is like the queen's envoy, traveling through your bloodstream, waiting to be converted into the active form, Free T3. Free T3 is the hormone that actually gets things done, powering your metabolism and keeping your energy levels up. If Free T4 levels are low, it usually means your thyroid isn't producing enough hormones, pointing towards hypothyroidism. High Free T4 levels can indicate hyperthyroidism, where your thyroid is in overdrive.

Then there's Free T3, the active form of thyroid hormone. Free T3 is like the queen's secret weapon, delivering the final, powerful punch. Low Free T3 levels can make you feel sluggish and tired, while high levels can leave you feeling jittery and anxious. Finally, we have Reverse T3. This is a bit like the queen's mischievous cousin getting in the way and blocking the effects of Free T3. High levels of Reverse T3 can contribute to symptoms of hypothyroidism, even if your other thyroid hormone levels appear normal.

Interpreting your thyroid blood panel results can feel like deciphering a foreign language, but it's not as complicated as it seems. Normal ranges for TSH are typically between 0.5 to 5.0 mIU/L, but optimal ranges might be narrower, depending on your symptoms. And depending on what standard of reference ranges your doctor uses or the lab where your blood work is done can differ. High TSH and low T4 levels are red flags for hypothyroidism, while low TSH and high T4 levels point towards hyperthyroidism. It's important to compare your TSH levels with your T3 and T4 levels to get a clearer picture of your thyroid health. Don't rely solely on TSH levels; Free T3 and Reverse T3 are equally important in understanding what's going on.

Common pitfalls in reading thyroid blood panels can lead to misdiagnosis or inadequate treatment. One major pitfall is relying solely on TSH levels. While TSH is a crucial marker, it doesn't tell the whole story. Your Free T3 and Reverse T3 levels provide additional insights into your thyroid function. Another common misconception is assuming that "normal" lab ranges mean everything is fine. Even if your levels fall within the normal range, you might still experience symptoms if they're not in the optimal range for you.

Knowing when to retest your thyroid levels is also essential for accurate diagnosis and effective treatment. After starting or adjusting medication, it's typically recommended to retest your levels in about six weeks to see how your body responds. Regular monitoring is crucial, especially if you're experiencing symptoms. Most doctors recommend checking your thyroid levels every three to six months to ensure your treatment plan is working effectively.

Understanding your thyroid blood panel can empower you to take control of your health. Knowing what each component measures and how to interpret the results, you can work more effectively with your healthcare provider to manage your thyroid condition. So, next time you're sitting in that doctor's office, waiting for your results, remember—you've got this! You're not just a passive patient; you're an informed advocate for your own health.

SELF-ASSESSMENT TOOLS: GAUGING YOUR THYROID HEALTH

Ever feel like you're on a never-ending rollercoaster of fatigue, mood swings, and brain fog? You're not alone; fortunately, you don't need a medical degree to start figuring out what's going on with your thyroid. Self-assessment tools can provide valuable insights and help you understand your symptoms better.

First up, let's talk about symptom checklists. These are your first line of defense in understanding what might be going on with your thyroid. Physical symptoms often include unrelenting fatigue that no amount of coffee can fix, unexplained weight gain or loss, and changes in your skin texture or hair thickness. Emotional symptoms might manifest as mood swings, depression, or heightened anxiety. Cognitive symptoms, like brain fog and memory issues, can make you feel like you're in a constant haze. Keeping a detailed checklist of these symptoms can help you identify patterns and provide a clearer picture to your healthcare provider.

Next, let's explore the basal body temperature method. This technique involves measuring your body temperature first thing in the morning before you even get out of bed. You'll need a reliable thermometer for this—preferably a digital one for accuracy. Place the thermometer under your tongue and keep it there until it beeps. Do this for several consecutive mornings to get an average reading. Women with thyroid issues often have consistently low body temperatures, usually below 97.8°F. If your temperatures are low, it could be a sign that your thyroid is underactive. Interpreting these temperature patterns can give you a preliminary indication of thyroid dysfunction, but following up with more comprehensive tests is important.

At-home test kits have become increasingly popular and can be a convenient way to check your thyroid health without making a trip to the doctor's office. Brands like LetsGetChecked and Everlywell offer reliable kits that measure key thyroid hormones like TSH, Free T4, and Free T3. When choosing a kit, look for one that includes a comprehensive panel. Collection is straightforward: you typically prick your finger to collect a small blood sample, which you then mail to a lab for analysis. Results usually return in a week or so, and many companies offer consultations with healthcare professionals to help you understand the results.

Journaling might sound old-fashioned, but keeping a daily health log can be incredibly useful. Start by tracking your energy levels, mood, and physical symptoms daily. A simple template can include columns for date, energy level (on a scale of 1-10), mood, and any notable symptoms like fatigue, weight changes, or cognitive issues. Over time, this log can reveal patterns and help you correlate symptoms with diet, lifestyle changes, and even medication adjustments. For instance, you might notice that your energy levels dip after eating certain foods or that your mood improves on days when you exercise. There is also a variety of health and wellness journals on the web that you can shop for, make your own on a spreadsheet, or just take notes in a notebook about your symptoms. Over time, this can help you and your healthcare provider make more informed decisions about your treatment plan.

Understanding your thyroid health doesn't have to be overwhelming. You can gain valuable insights and take proactive steps in managing your thyroid by using symptom checklists, basal body temperature measurements, at-home test kits, and daily health logs. These tools can provide a clearer picture of your health and help you communicate more effectively with your healthcare provider.

FINDING THE RIGHT HEALTHCARE PROVIDER: ADVOCATE FOR YOURSELF

Finding the right healthcare provider to diagnose and treat your thyroid condition is like finding the perfect hairstylist—you need someone who understands you, listens to your needs, and has the skills to get the job done right. Different types of specialists can help with thyroid conditions, and knowing who to turn to can make all the difference.

Endocrinologists are the go-to experts when it comes to thyroid health. They specialize in the endocrine system, which includes glands like the thyroid, pituitary, and adrenal glands. If you're dealing with a complex thyroid disorder or need specialized care, an endocrinologist is your best bet. They have the expertise to handle everything from hypothyroidism and hyperthyroidism to thyroid nodules and cancer. Sometimes, you can just call an endocrinologist's office and request an appointment. Most often, you usually have to have a referral from your PCP, but if your PCP keeps telling you your blood work is within normal range, they have no reason to refer you to an endocrinologist. Which is why I recommend seeking out a functional doctor if your PCP won't refer you to an endocrinologists because they see no reason to since your blood work is within "normal range".

Functional medicine practitioners take a holistic approach to health, focusing on identifying and addressing the root causes of disease. They often spend more time with their patients and consider factors like diet, lifestyle, and environmental exposures. A functional medicine practitioner might be the right fit if you're looking for a more comprehensive and integrative approach to managing your thyroid health.

Integrative health specialists combine conventional medicine with alternative therapies, offering a balanced approach to treatment. They might incorporate acupuncture, herbal medicine, and nutritional counseling into your care plan. This type of specialist can be particularly helpful if you're interested in exploring natural remedies alongside traditional treatments.

Evaluating the credentials and experience of healthcare providers is crucial for ensuring you're in good hands. Start by checking for board certifications, which indicate that the provider has completed specialized training and passed rigorous exams in their field. Specializations in thyroid health are a bonus, showing that the provider has focused expertise in managing thyroid conditions. Patient reviews and testimonials can also offer valuable insights. Look for feedback on their bedside manner, communication skills, and overall effectiveness.

Preparing for medical appointments can make a difference in how productive those visits are. Start by creating a list of symptoms and questions. Write down everything, even if it seems minor. This helps ensure you don't forget anything important during the appointment. Bring previous medical records, including past blood test results and imaging studies. This provides context and helps your healthcare provider make informed decisions about your care. Discuss your treatment preferences openly. If you prefer natural remedies or specific medications, let your provider know. This sets the stage for a collaborative relationship where your needs and preferences are prioritized.

Effective communication with your healthcare provider is key to advocating for your health. Don't be afraid to ask for comprehensive testing. If you feel that your symptoms are being dismissed or not fully addressed, insist on a full thyroid panel that includes TSH, Free T4, Free T3, and Reverse T3. Express your concerns and preferences clearly. Use statements like, "I've noticed these symptoms, and I'm worried about how they're affecting my daily life," or "I prefer a more natural approach to treatment; what are my options?" This ensures your voice is heard and your needs are considered.

Seeking second opinions is sometimes necessary, especially if you feel uncertain about a diagnosis or treatment plan. Don't hesitate to get another perspective if something doesn't sit right with you. It's your health, and you deserve to feel confident in your care. Remember, a good healthcare provider will respect your decision to seek additional opinions and will support you in finding the best path forward.

Navigating the healthcare system can be daunting, but finding the right provider and advocating for yourself can lead to better outcomes and a more satisfying care experience. Whether you're working with an endocrinologist, a functional medicine practitioner, or an integrative health specialist, the goal is to find someone who listens to you, understands your needs, and partners with you on your journey to better thyroid health.

COMMON MISDIAGNOSES: WHEN IT'S NOT JUST IN YOUR HEAD

Ever felt like you're living in a fog, only to be told it's "just stress" or "part of aging"? You're not alone. Many women find themselves misdiagnosed with conditions that mimic thyroid disorders. One of the most common culprits is chronic fatigue syndrome (CFS). People with CFS experience overwhelming fatigue that doesn't improve with rest and worsens with physical or mental activity. Sound familiar? It's easy to see how this could be mistaken for thyroid issues, especially when fatigue is a hallmark symptom of both conditions.

Depression and anxiety disorders are also frequently confused with thyroid problems. When you're dealing with mood swings, irritability, and a general sense of malaise, it's tempting for both you and your doctor to chalk it up to mental health. But what if there's more to the story? Depression can make you feel sluggish and unmotivated, while anxiety can cause palpitations and a sense of unease—symptoms that are also common in thyroid disorders. Menopausal symptoms further complicate the picture, bringing their own set of challenges like hot flashes, night sweats, and mood changes. These symptoms overlap significantly with thyroid dysfunction, making it easy to misdiagnose.

Differentiating thyroid symptoms from these other conditions requires a keen eye and a bit of detective work. One way to distinguish them is by looking at the unique combination of symptoms. For example, while both depression and hypothyroidism can cause fatigue and weight gain, hypothyroidism often comes with additional symptoms like dry skin, hair loss, and cold intolerance. The duration and progression of symptoms can also provide clues. Thyroid-related symptoms often develop gradually and persist despite lifestyle changes, whereas symptoms from conditions like CFS or depression might fluctuate more noticeably with stress levels or environmental changes.

Consider Breanna's story. She was initially diagnosed with depression after experiencing extreme fatigue, weight gain, and mood swings. Her doctor prescribed antidepressants, but Breanna didn't feel any better. Frustrated, she sought a second opinion and insisted on a full thyroid panel. Lo and behold, her TSH levels were through the roof, indicating hypothyroidism. With the right medication, Breanna's symptoms improved dramatically. Then there's Melanie, who struggled with chronic fatigue for years. Doctors told her it was just stress, but she knew something was off. After pushing for comprehensive testing, she was finally diagnosed with hypothyroidism. Medication and lifestyle changes transformed her life, putting an end to years of frustration.

Advocating for comprehensive testing is crucial for an accurate diagnosis. Don't settle for a basic TSH test. Insist on a full thyroid panel that includes Free T4, Free T3, and Reverse T3. These tests provide a more complete picture of your thyroid function and can reveal issues that a simple TSH test might miss. Additional tests for thyroid antibodies can help diagnose autoimmune conditions like Hashimoto's or Graves' disease. Imaging studies, such as thyroid ultrasounds, can detect nodules or structural abnormalities that might be contributing to your symptoms.

The importance of thorough evaluations cannot be overstated. If your symptoms persist despite normal lab results, don't be afraid to push for more tests or seek a second opinion. Your healthcare provider should be your partner in this process, helping you navigate the complexities of thyroid health. Remember, it's your body, and you know it best. Trust your instincts and advocate for the care you deserve.

By understanding the common misdiagnoses and how to differentiate thyroid symptoms, you can take proactive steps toward getting the right diagnosis and treatment. Whether it's chronic fatigue, depression, anxiety, or menopausal symptoms, don't let misdiagnoses keep you from feeling your best. The proper tests and a healthcare provider who listens can make all the difference.

TRACKING YOUR PROGRESS: KEEPING TABS ON YOUR HEALTH

Imagine you've just started a new thyroid medication. You're hopeful but also a bit skeptical. How do you know if it's working? This is where regular monitoring comes in. Keeping tabs on your thyroid health is crucial for adjusting treatment plans and catching any changes early. Think of it as a way to fine-tune your body, like adjusting the strings on a guitar to get the perfect sound. By regularly monitoring your symptoms and lab results, you can ensure that your treatment is effective and make adjustments as needed. Detecting changes early can prevent your condition from worsening and help you maintain a better quality of life.

In today's tech-savvy world, plenty of tools and apps are designed to help you track your thyroid health. Health tracking apps like MyFitnessPal or Apple Health can be incredibly useful. These apps allow you to log your symptoms, medication, diet, and exercise routines all in one place. They can even send reminders to take your medication or schedule your next doctor's appointment. Digital health journals are another great option. Apps like Bearable or Guava: Health Tracker offer secure, easy-to-use platforms where you can document your daily health status. These tools make it easier to spot patterns and correlations that you might miss otherwise, giving you a clearer picture of your overall health.

Interpreting changes in your symptoms and lab results can feel like solving a complex puzzle, but it's more straightforward than it seems. Start by correlating symptom improvements with your lab results. For instance, if you notice that your energy levels are rising and your brain fog is lifting, check your latest thyroid panel. Are your TSH levels within the optimal range? Are your Free T4 and Free T3 levels balanced? Recognizing when to seek medical advice is also crucial. If your symptoms persist or worsen despite normal lab results, it's time to consult your healthcare provider. They might need to adjust your medication or explore other underlying issues.

Adjusting your lifestyle and treatment plans based on tracking results is a proactive way to manage your thyroid health. Modifying your diet and exercise routines can have a significant impact. If you notice that certain foods trigger symptoms, consider eliminating them from your diet. Likewise, incorporating thyroid-friendly foods like selenium-rich Brazil nuts or iodine-rich seaweed can support your thyroid function. Exercise is another key player. Regular physical activity can help regulate your metabolism and improve your mood. Discussing medication adjustments with your healthcare provider is also essential. If your lab results indicate that your current dosage isn't effective, your provider might recommend increasing or decreasing your medication.

Celebrating small victories and maintaining motivation are equally important. Managing a thyroid condition can be a long and sometimes frustrating process, but acknowledging your progress can make a big difference. Did you manage to exercise three times this week? Celebrate that! Did you notice an improvement in your energy levels? Give yourself a pat on the back. Keeping a positive mindset and celebrating these small wins can help you stay motivated and committed to your treatment plan.

Regular monitoring and tracking can empower you to take control of your thyroid health. You can manage your condition more effectively by using tools and apps to log your symptoms and lab results, interpreting changes, and making informed adjustments to your lifestyle and treatment plans. Remember, you're not just a passive patient; you're an active participant in your own health journey.

As we wrap up this chapter, remember that tracking your progress is like having a roadmap for your thyroid health. It helps you see where you've been, where you are, and where you're headed. With the right tools and a proactive approach, you can navigate the complexities of thyroid health and feel more in control. Up next, we'll explore natural remedies and lifestyle changes that can further support your thyroid and overall well-being.

5

THE QUEEN'S ALLIES: THE GUT-THYROID CONNECTION IN HER ROYAL COURT

Let's embark on a journey to a fascinating part of your body: Your gut. Picture your gut as a bustling medieval marketplace, with vendors shouting their wares, townsfolk milling about, and the occasional thief sneaking through the crowd. Now, what if the walls of this marketplace started to crumble, letting all sorts of undesirables slip through? That's essentially what happens in your gut when you have leaky gut syndrome. The walls of your intestines, which should be tight and secure, develop tiny cracks and holes, allowing toxins, bacteria, and undigested food particles to pass into your bloodstream. This, my friend, is where the intrigue of understanding your gut as a complex system begins.

LEAKY GUT: HOW IT AFFECTS YOUR THYROID

So, what exactly is leaky gut syndrome? It's a condition where the lining of your intestines becomes more permeable than it should be. Normally, your gut lining is like a tightly guarded castle wall, keeping out invaders while letting in only the good stuff—nutrients and water. This integrity is maintained by structures called tight junctions, which are like the gatekeepers ensuring no riffraff gets through. However, when these tight junctions become loose, it's as if the castle gates are left ajar, allowing toxins and other harmful substances to slip through.

Several factors can contribute to a leaky gut. Chronic stress is a big one. When you're stressed, your body produces cortisol, which can weaken the gut lining over time. A poor diet, especially one high in processed foods, sugar, and alcohol, can also damage the gut lining. These foods can inflame the gut and disrupt the balance of good and bad bacteria, further compromising gut integrity. Other culprits include infections, medications like antibiotics and NSAIDs, and even nutrient deficiencies.

When your gut becomes leaky, it triggers an inflammatory response. Your immune system, the vigilant guardian of your body, sees the toxins and undigested food particles as invaders and launches an attack. This chronic inflammation can affect various parts of your body, including your thyroid. In fact, there's a significant connection between leaky gut and autoimmune thyroid diseases like Hashimoto's thyroiditis. The constant inflammation can cause your immune system to go haywire, leading it to mistakenly attack your thyroid gland.

When toxins and undigested food particles enter your bloodstream, they can trigger autoimmune reactions. For instance, gluten, a protein found in wheat, barley, and rye, can be particularly problematic. In some people, gluten can cause the release of a protein called zonulin, which increases gut permeability. This can lead to a vicious cycle of inflammation and autoimmunity, making conditions like Hashimoto's worse. It's like having a mole in your kingdom, constantly undermining your defenses.

So, how do you know if you have a leaky gut? The symptoms can be varied and often overlap with other conditions. Chronic fatigue and low energy are common complaints. You might always feel tired, no matter how much sleep you get. Digestive issues like bloating, gas, and irregular bowel movements are also telltale signs. Food sensitivities and allergies can develop or worsen, making you react to foods that never bothered you before. Joint pain and skin issues like eczema and rashes can also be linked to leaky gut. It's like your body is sending out distress signals, trying to tell you something's not right. Being self-aware and proactive in identifying these symptoms can empower you to take control of your health.

Healing a leaky gut involves several strategies. First, consider eliminating trigger foods from your diet. Gluten and dairy are common culprits, so try cutting them out for a few weeks to see if your symptoms improve (That was the hardest thing for me to do since I love dairy foods, pasta, and bread. It took me a month just to mentally prepare myself for that strategy. But remember, these are only suggestions, not a mandate. It's your body and your health, and you can decide how to improve your health.) Incorporating gut-healing foods is also crucial. Bone broth is a fantastic option as it's rich in collagen and amino acids that help repair the gut lining. Fermented foods like sauerkraut, kimchi, and yogurt can introduce beneficial bacteria to help restore balance in your gut.

Supplements can also support gut healing. L-glutamine is an amino acid that helps repair the gut lining. Collagen supplements can also be beneficial, providing the building blocks your gut needs to heal. Stress management is another essential component. Techniques like mindfulness meditation, deep breathing exercises (I know I am starting to sound like a broken record, but stress management is the key foundation to your health), and just getting out in nature for walks can help reduce stress and support overall gut health.

Leaky Gut Healing Checklist

1. Eliminate Trigger Foods: Cut out gluten, dairy, and processed foods for 2-3 weeks.
2. Incorporate Gut-Healing Foods: Add bone broth, fermented foods, and fiber-rich vegetables to your diet.
3. Use Supportive Supplements: Consider L-glutamine and collagen to aid gut repair.
4. Manage Stress: Practice mindfulness, yoga, or other relaxation techniques like walking.

By addressing these factors, you can help repair your gut lining and reduce inflammation, giving your thyroid a better chance to function optimally. Healing your gut is like fortifying your castle walls, ensuring that no unwanted invaders can disrupt the peace in your kingdom.

GUT MICROBIOME: THE HIDDEN FACTOR IN THYROID HEALTH

Imagine your gut as a bustling city with trillions of tiny inhabitants, all working together to keep things running smoothly. This bustling metropolis is your gut microbiome, a diverse microbial community that calls your intestines home. These microscopic residents play a crucial role in your overall health, helping with digestion, producing vitamins, and keeping your immune system in check. It's like having an army of tiny workers ensuring everything functions as it should. The balance between beneficial and harmful bacteria is vital. When this balance is disrupted, it can lead to a host of health issues, including problems with your thyroid.

The gut microbiome has a significant impact on thyroid health. One of its critical roles involves the conversion of thyroid hormones. Your thyroid produces T4, which is then converted into the more active T3 in various tissues, including the gut. Healthy gut bacteria aid this conversion process, ensuring you have enough active thyroid hormone to keep your metabolism and energy levels up. However, when the balance of bacteria is off—a condition known as dysbiosis—this conversion can be impaired. Dysbiosis can lead to increased inflammation and even trigger autoimmune responses, exacerbating conditions like Hashimoto's thyroiditis.

An imbalanced gut microbiome, or dysbiosis, can manifest in various ways. Frequent digestive issues, such as bloating, diarrhea, and gas, are common signs that your gut bacteria are out of whack. You might also experience persistent fatigue and brain fog, making it hard to concentrate or stay alert during the day. Unexplained weight changes, either gaining or losing weight without any significant changes to your diet or activity levels, can also point to a gut imbalance. Skin problems like acne, eczema, and recurring infections are other indicators that your gut might need some attention. These symptoms are your body's way of waving a red flag, signaling that something isn't right.

Supporting a healthy gut microbiome involves several actionable steps. First, focus on incorporating diverse, fiber-rich foods into your diet. Fruits, vegetables, legumes, and whole grains provide the fiber that beneficial bacteria thrive on. Reducing your intake of sugar and processed foods is also crucial. These foods can feed harmful bacteria and yeast, tipping the balance in the wrong direction. Prebiotic and probiotic supplements can help restore and maintain a healthy gut flora. Prebiotics are the food that nourishes your good bacteria, while probiotics are the beneficial bacteria themselves. Including fermented foods like yogurt, kimchi, kombucha, and sauerkraut can provide a natural source of probiotics, further supporting your gut health.

Gut Health Support Tips

1. Incorporate Fiber-Rich Foods: Add plenty of fruits, vegetables, legumes, and whole grains to your meals.
2. Reduce Sugar and Processed Foods: Limit sweets, sodas, and packaged snacks.
3. Use Prebiotic and Probiotic Supplements: Look for high-quality options to boost your gut flora.
4. Include Fermented Foods: Enjoy yogurt, kimchi, sauerkraut, and other fermented goodies regularly.

By taking these steps, you can help restore balance to your gut microbiome, supporting your digestive health and thyroid function.

PROBIOTICS AND PREBIOTICS: FEEDING YOUR GUT FOR BETTER THYROID FUNCTION

Back to your gut as a bustling city, with probiotics as the friendly residents keeping everything running smoothly. Probiotics are live beneficial bacteria that help maintain balance in your gut. Think of them as the good guys who fend off harmful invaders. You can find probiotics in supplements or fermented foods like yogurt, sauerkraut, kombucha and kefir. Prebiotics, on the other hand, are the food that these good bacteria thrive on. They are like the nutritious soil that helps plants grow. Prebiotics are found in fiber-rich vegetables, legumes, and whole grains. So, while probiotics are the beneficial bacteria, prebiotics are the sustenance that keeps them flourishing.

When it comes to thyroid health, probiotics play a crucial role. They enhance gut barrier integrity, ensuring that your gut lining remains strong and impermeable. This is important because a compromised gut can lead to inflammation, triggering autoimmune responses and exacerbating conditions like Hashimoto's thyroiditis. By maintaining a healthy gut barrier, probiotics help reduce inflammation and support your immune system. Additionally, probiotics aid in nutrient absorption and metabolism. A healthy gut ensures that your body efficiently absorbs essential nutrients like iodine, selenium, and zinc, which are vital for thyroid function. By supporting your gut health, probiotics indirectly support your thyroid, helping you maintain optimal energy levels and overall well-being.

Prebiotics are equally important for gut and thyroid health. They promote the growth of beneficial bacteria in your gut, creating a thriving environment for probiotics. Prebiotics also enhance the production of short-chain fatty acids (SCFAs), which play a key role in maintaining gut health and regulating inflammation. SCFAs help strengthen the gut lining and support immune function, reducing the risk of autoimmune reactions that can affect the thyroid. By feeding the good bacteria in your gut, prebiotics help maintain a balanced microbiome, which is crucial for overall health.

Incorporating probiotics and prebiotics into your diet is simpler than you might think. Start by adding fermented foods and drinks like sauerkraut, kefir, kombucha, and miso to your meals. These foods are rich in probiotics and can help boost your gut health. Including prebiotic-rich foods like asparagus, garlic, onions, and bananas can provide the nourishment your beneficial bacteria need to thrive. When choosing probiotic supplements, look for high-quality options that contain a variety of strains and a substantial number of colony-forming units (CFUs). This ensures you're getting a diverse and potent dose of beneficial bacteria. Finally, aim to create balanced meals that support gut health by combining probiotics and prebiotics. For example, a salad with mixed greens, garlic, and a side of fermented veggies can be both delicious and gut-friendly.

By making these dietary changes, you can support your gut health, which in turn supports your thyroid. It's like giving your body the tools it needs to maintain balance and function optimally.

DIGESTIVE ENZYMES AND THYROID HEALTH: A SYMBIOTIC RELATIONSHIP

Picture this: you've just enjoyed a delicious meal, but soon after, you're feeling bloated and gassy. What gives? Enter digestive enzymes, your body's unsung heroes that break down proteins, fats, and carbohydrates into nutrients you can actually use. These enzymes come from various sources, primarily your pancreas and stomach. Think of them as tiny workers, each with a specific job—breaking down a steak into amino acids, turning a slice of butter into fatty acids, and converting a piece of bread into simple sugars. Without these hardworking enzymes, your body would struggle to absorb and utilize nutrients, leaving you feeling less than fabulous.

So, how do digestive enzymes impact your thyroid? It's all about nutrient absorption. To produce hormones, your thyroid needs certain nutrients, like iodine, selenium, and zinc. When digestive enzymes aren't doing their job, you might end up with nutrient deficiencies. This can compromise thyroid hormone production and lead to symptoms like fatigue, weight gain, and brain fog. It's like trying to bake a cake without key ingredients; you won't get the desired result. Poor digestion can also lead to malabsorption of thyroid medications, making them less effective. If your body can't properly break down and absorb these meds, they can't do their job of regulating your thyroid function.

How do you know if you're lacking in digestive enzymes? There are several telltale signs. Bloating and gas after meals are common symptoms. If you find yourself feeling like a balloon ready to pop after eating, it could be a sign your enzymes need a boost. Undigested food in your stools is another indicator. If you notice pieces of food in your waste, it means your body isn't breaking down food properly. Nutrient deficiencies can manifest as hair loss, brittle nails, or even anemia. Frequent indigestion and heartburn are also red flags. If you're constantly popping antacids, it might be time to examine your enzyme levels.

Improving your enzyme function can make a world of difference. Start by incorporating enzyme-rich foods into your diet. Pineapple and papaya are fantastic options as they contain natural enzymes like bromelain and papain, which help break down proteins. Digestive enzyme supplements can also be beneficial. Look for high-quality supplements that contain a blend of enzymes to aid in the digestion of proteins, fats, and carbohydrates. Chewing your food thoroughly is another simple yet effective strategy. The process of chewing signals your body to start producing digestive enzymes, making the entire digestive process more efficient.

It is also crucial to avoid the overuse of antacids and other medications that impair enzyme function. While antacids can provide temporary relief, they can disrupt the production of stomach acid, which is essential for enzyme activity. Instead of relying on antacids, consider natural remedies for heartburn and indigestion, like ginger tea or apple cider vinegar. These can help soothe your stomach without compromising enzyme function.

By paying attention to your digestive health and supporting your enzyme function, you can improve nutrient absorption, enhance the efficacy of your thyroid medications, and reduce unpleasant symptoms like bloating and gas. It's all about giving your body the tools it needs to function at its best. So, next time you sit down for a meal, remember those tiny workers in your gut and give them a little extra support. Your thyroid will thank you.

HEALING YOUR GUT: DIETARY AND LIFESTYLE CHANGES

When it comes to gut health, your diet plays a starring role. Think of it as the foundation of a sturdy house. Without a solid base, everything else crumbles. A gut-healing diet focuses on anti-inflammatory foods that soothe and repair your digestive tract. Inflammation is the enemy here, often causing or exacerbating gut issues. Foods rich in omega-3 fatty acids, like salmon and chia seeds, are excellent anti-inflammatories. They help calm the gut and reduce systemic inflammation, which can also benefit your thyroid. Avoiding processed and high-sugar foods is equally crucial. These foods can irritate the gut lining and feed harmful bacteria, creating a vicious cycle of inflammation and imbalance. Instead, prioritize nutrient-dense, whole foods like fresh fruits, vegetables, lean proteins, and whole grains. These foods provide the vitamins, minerals, and fiber your gut needs to function optimally.

Specific dietary choices can make a significant difference in healing your gut. Bone broth is a fantastic option for repairing the gut lining. It's rich in collagen and gelatin, which help strengthen the intestinal walls. Fermented foods like kimchi, sauerkraut, and yogurt introduce beneficial bacteria into your gut, supporting a healthy microbiome. Fiber-rich vegetables, such as broccoli, Brussels sprouts, and artichokes, act as prebiotics, feeding the good bacteria. Omega-3-rich foods, like flaxseeds, walnuts, and fatty fish, offer anti-inflammatory benefits that support both gut and thyroid health. Incorporating these foods into your diet can create a gut-friendly environment that promotes healing and balance.

Lifestyle changes play an equally important role in maintaining gut integrity. Regular physical activity is a game-changer. Exercise helps keep your digestive system moving and reduces stress, which can otherwise wreak havoc on your gut. Managing stress through mindfulness and relaxation techniques is another key factor. Chronic stress can weaken the gut lining, so practices like meditation, deep breathing, and yoga can be incredibly beneficial. Ensuring you get enough sleep is crucial for gut recovery. Your body does a lot of its repair work while you sleep, so aim for 7-9 hours of quality rest each night. Together, these lifestyle changes support a healthy gut, which in turn supports your overall well-being.

Healing your gut doesn't happen overnight, but a structured plan can help you stay on track. Start with an elimination phase, removing common trigger foods like gluten, dairy, and processed sugars from your diet. This phase lasts about 4-6 weeks, allowing your gut to heal without the constant barrage of irritants. Next, move to the reintroduction phase, where you slowly add back foods one at a time to see how your body reacts. This helps identify specific food sensitivities. Finally, enter the maintenance phase, where you stick to a balanced diet and healthy lifestyle habits long-term. Regularly monitor your progress and adjust as needed, keeping an eye on how your gut—and, by extension, your thyroid—responds. This comprehensive approach ensures that you're not just putting a band-aid on the problem but addressing it at its root.

Step-by-Step Gut Healing Plan

1. Elimination Phase: Remove gluten, dairy, and processed sugars for 4-6 weeks.
2. Reintroduction Phase: Gradually add back foods to identify sensitivities.
3. Maintenance Phase: Adopt long-term dietary and lifestyle habits.
4. Monitor Progress: Keep track of your symptoms and adjust as needed.

By following these steps, you can create a gut environment that supports healing and overall health. Remember, your gut and thyroid are intricately connected, and taking care of one helps the other. As you make these changes, you'll likely notice improvements not just in your digestion but in your energy levels, mood, and overall well-being. It's all about giving your body the support it needs to thrive.

In this chapter, we've explored the powerful connection between gut and thyroid health, exploring how diet, probiotics, prebiotics, and lifestyle changes can make a real difference. Up next, we'll delve into the role of the pituitary gland—a small but mighty player in the thyroid's world. Stay tuned for more insights that will help you take control of your health and well-being.

THANK YOU

Dear Reader,

Thank you so much for taking the time to read *The Small but Mighty Thyroid: Meet Your Tiny Queen of Health and Energy*. I truly hope that this book has provided you with valuable insights into the often-overlooked role the thyroid plays in your overall health. Whether you're just beginning your journey to better thyroid health or deepening your understanding, I hope the information was both empowering and practical.

Your thyroid might be small, but as you've learned, its impact on your body is immense. My goal was to help you connect the dots, understand symptoms, and feel confident in managing your thyroid health with knowledge and care. Whether it's through lifestyle changes, understanding test results, or working with healthcare providers, every step you take towards better thyroid health is significant.

I'd love to hear your thoughts!

If *The Small but Mighty Thyroid* has helped you, even in a small way, would you mind sharing your experience in an honest review on Amazon? Your feedback helps other readers discover the book and gives me the opportunity to improve and continue creating content that matters. Whether you share how the book made things clearer for you or what specific information stood out, I'd deeply appreciate your review.

How to Leave a Review

Leaving a review is simple and only takes a few minutes. Scan the QR code Below to leave your review.

Thank you again for your time, trust, and for being a part of this journey. Your review means the world to me and will help others on their path to better thyroid health.

With gratitude,

Tiffany Rose

6

THE QUEEN'S COMMAND: BALANCING HORMONES TO SUPPORT THYROID HEALTH

Imagine you're the conductor of a grand orchestra. Every instrument needs to be in perfect harmony for the symphony to sound just right. Now, replace the orchestra with your hormones, and you've got a pretty accurate picture of what's happening inside your body. When one hormone is out of tune, it can throw off the entire performance, and your thyroid is no exception. Let's dive into the fascinating world of hormones and how they interact with your thyroid.

THE HORMONE-THYROID LINK: UNDERSTANDING THE CONNECTION

First, let's get to know the endocrine system, the unsung hero of your body's hormone regulation. It's like the backstage crew at a rock concert, ensuring everything runs smoothly. The major players include the pituitary gland, thyroid, adrenal glands, and ovaries. These glands produce hormones that act as messengers, telling your body what to do and when to do it. The pituitary gland, often called the "master gland," is like the stage manager, orchestrating the release of hormones from other glands. It produces thyroid-stimulating hormone (TSH), which tells your thyroid to produce T3 and T4, the hormones that regulate your metabolism. The adrenal glands produce cortisol, your body's main stress hormone, while the ovaries produce estrogen and progesterone, which regulate your menstrual cycle and reproductive health.

The endocrine system works through a series of feedback loops, much like a thermostat controlling the temperature in your home. When your body senses that thyroid hormone levels are low, the pituitary gland releases TSH to stimulate the thyroid. Once the thyroid produces enough hormones, the pituitary gland gets the signal to stop releasing TSH. This hormonal hierarchy and feedback loop ensure that everything stays in balance—most of the time.

Thyroid hormones don't work in isolation. They interact with other key hormones to keep your body functioning optimally. Take estrogen and progesterone, for example. These hormones have a significant impact on thyroid function. Estrogen increases thyroid-binding globulin (TBG) levels, a protein that carries thyroid hormones in your blood. When there's too much estrogen, it can lead to higher levels of TBG, which means less free thyroid hormone is available for your body to use. This is why estrogen dominance can make thyroid symptoms worse. Progesterone, on the other hand, helps balance the effects of estrogen and supports thyroid hormone utilization.

Then there's cortisol, the stress hormone. When you're stressed, your adrenal glands pump out cortisol like it's going out of style. High levels of cortisol can interfere with the conversion of T4 to T3, the active form of thyroid hormone. This can leave you feeling sluggish and tired despite having normal T4 levels. Insulin, the hormone that regulates blood sugar, also plays a role. Insulin resistance, a condition where your body's cells don't respond normally to insulin, can affect your thyroid by increasing inflammation and disrupting hormone production.

Let's look at some real-life examples to illustrate these interactions. Meet Laura, a 42-year-old woman who started experiencing fatigue, weight gain, and mood swings. Her doctor discovered that she had estrogen dominance, which was increasing her levels of TBG and reducing the amount of free thyroid hormone available for her body to use. By addressing her estrogen dominance through dietary changes and supplements, Laura was able to balance her hormones and improve her thyroid function.

Now, let's talk about stress. Paige, a high-powered executive, found herself constantly stressed out from work. Her cortisol levels were through the roof, and she started experiencing symptoms of hypothyroidism. Her doctor explained that the high cortisol levels were interfering with her thyroid hormone conversion. By incorporating stress management techniques like mindfulness meditation, yoga, regular exercise, spending time in nature, and maintaining a healthy work-life balance, Paige was able to lower her cortisol levels and improve her thyroid function.

Understanding the intricate dance between your thyroid hormones and other hormones is crucial for managing your thyroid health. By addressing imbalances in estrogen, progesterone, cortisol, and insulin, you can support your thyroid and improve your overall well-being. This holistic approach ensures that your body's symphony plays in perfect harmony, allowing you to feel your best.

MANAGING HORMONAL FLUCTUATIONS: TIPS FOR PERIMENOPAUSAL WOMEN

As you enter your late 40s, you may find your body embarking on a rollercoaster ride of hormonal fluctuations you didn't sign up for. Welcome to perimenopause, a phase where understanding these changes can empower you to navigate this journey with confidence. Your estrogen and progesterone levels start to decline, and your once-predictable menstrual cycles become a game of roulette. One month, you're early; the next, you're late; sometimes, you skip altogether. These hormonal changes bring along a host of symptoms, like hot flashes that make you feel like you're roasting from the inside out and night sweats that leave you waking up drenched.

Now, let's talk about how these hormonal shifts affect your thyroid. It's important to understand that perimenopause can exacerbate thyroid issues you might already be dealing with. As your estrogen levels drop, it can lead to an increased incidence of hypothyroidism. You might find that your fatigue is worse, those extra pounds are even harder to shed, and your mood swings are rivaling those of a teenager. The tricky part is that many symptoms of perimenopause and thyroid dysfunction overlap, making diagnosis a bit of a challenge. But rest assured, you're not alone in this. Many women experience similar challenges, and understanding these hormonal fluctuations can help you feel reassured and understood.

So, what can you do to manage these hormonal fluctuations? You can take charge of your health by making simple yet effective changes to your lifestyle. Start with your diet. Phytoestrogen-rich foods like flaxseeds and soy products can help balance your hormones naturally. These plant-based compounds mimic estrogen in your body, providing some relief from those pesky symptoms. Herbal supplements like black cohosh and red clover have been shown to help with hot flashes and mood swings. Regular physical activity is another game-changer. Exercise helps balance your hormones, reduce stress, and improve your overall mood. You don't have to become a gym rat; even a daily walk can make a big difference. By incorporating these strategies into your life, you can feel proactive and in control of your hormonal health.

- Soy and soy products: Soybeans, tofu, miso soup, and miso paste are all high in isoflavones, a type of phytoestrogen.
- Nuts and seeds: Almonds, flaxseeds, peanuts, sesame seeds, sunflower seeds, and Brazil nuts are all high in phytoestrogens.
- Fruits: Apples, berries, grapes, peaches, pears, and plums all contain phytoestrogens.
- Vegetables: Broccoli, Brussels sprouts, kale, onions, spinach, sprouts, cabbage, garlic, and zucchini are all high in phytoestrogens.
- Grains: Barley, oats, and wheat germ all contain phytoestrogens.

Stress management techniques like yoga and meditation can also be incredibly beneficial. These practices help lower your cortisol levels, which can, in turn, improve your thyroid function. Imagine taking a yoga class where you finally get to exhale all that pent-up stress—blissful, right?

Let's look at some real-life success stories to inspire you. Meet Molly, a 50-year-old woman who was struggling with perimenopausal symptoms and hypothyroidism. She decided to make some lifestyle changes, starting with her diet. Linda added flaxseeds to her morning smoothie and incorporated soy products into her meals. She also started taking black cohosh supplements.

Within a few months, she noticed a significant improvement in her symptoms. Her hot flashes were less frequent, and her mood swings were more manageable.

Then there's Kristi, who was overwhelmed by fatigue and weight gain. She started practicing yoga and meditation daily, which helped her manage stress and improve her energy levels. Kristi also included phytoestrogen-rich foods in her diet and took red clover supplements. Over time, she saw an improvement in her thyroid function and felt more in control of her health.

These stories show that with the right strategies, you can manage perimenopausal symptoms and support your thyroid health. It's all about finding what works best for you and making small changes that add up to significant improvements. So, grab those flaxseeds, roll out your yoga mat, and take a step toward feeling like yourself again.

INSULIN RESISTANCE AND THYROID DYSFUNCTION: THE OVERLAP

Imagine your body as a factory, with insulin acting as the manager, directing glucose (sugar) into your cells to be used for energy. Insulin resistance happens when your cells stop listening to insulin's instructions, leaving glucose to float around in your bloodstream, causing high blood sugar. This condition often stems from a mix of factors such as a diet high in refined carbs and sugars, a sedentary lifestyle, and, yes, even your genes. If your family tree is dotted with diabetes or metabolic issues, you might be more prone to insulin resistance.

The connection between insulin resistance and thyroid dysfunction is like a tangled web. When your cells resist insulin, your body's metabolic rate can slow down, making you feel like you're constantly dragging. This impacts your thyroid because it can interfere with converting T4 (inactive thyroid hormone) to T3 (active thyroid hormone), which is crucial for maintaining your energy levels. Insulin resistance can also contribute to weight gain and make it harder to lose those stubborn pounds, creating a vicious cycle of metabolic mayhem.

What are the tell-tale signs of insulin resistance? For starters, persistent fatigue and low energy levels are common. You might find yourself craving sugary and high-carb foods, which only adds fuel to the fire. Abdominal weight gain is another red flag, as is the difficulty in shedding those extra pounds. If you've noticed your blood sugar and cholesterol levels creeping up, it could be a sign that insulin resistance is at play. These symptoms are your body's way of waving a red flag, signaling that something's off balance.

Managing insulin resistance involves a few strategic moves. Start with your diet. A low-glycemic diet rich in whole foods can help improve insulin sensitivity. Focus on foods that don't cause a spike in blood sugar, like vegetables, whole grains, and lean proteins. Regular physical activity, especially strength training, can also be a game-changer. Building muscle helps improve insulin sensitivity, making it easier for your cells to respond to insulin's instructions. Supplements like chromium and berberine have been shown to support blood sugar regulation and improve insulin sensitivity. Lastly, keep an eye on your blood sugar levels. Regular monitoring can help you track your progress and make necessary adjustments to your diet and lifestyle.

To make this more actionable, consider the following checklist for managing insulin resistance:

Insulin Resistance Management Checklist

1. Adopt a Low-Glycemic Diet: Focus on whole foods that don't spike blood sugar.
2. Engage in Regular Physical Activity: Incorporate strength training into your routine.
3. Use Supportive Supplements: Consider chromium and berberine for blood sugar regulation. *But remember to always check with your doctor before starting any supplements to make sure they don't interfere with any other medication you're on.*
4. Monitor Blood Sugar Levels: Keep track of your levels to make informed adjustments.

Using a Continuous Glucose Monitor (CGM) can be a valuable tool for keeping track of your blood sugar levels in real-time. Unlike traditional finger-prick methods, a CGM provides continuous updates, offering insights into how food, exercise, stress, and hormones impact daily glucose levels. This is especially important for women, as hormonal fluctuations during the menstrual cycle, pregnancy, perimenopause, or menopause can cause significant changes in blood sugar. With a CGM, you can make timely adjustments to your diet, lifestyle, or medications, helping you maintain better overall health and hormonal balance. Lots of women also like using the CMG periodically to learn what foods spike their insulin and by how much.

Another way to see where you stand on the insulin resistance path is to check your hemoglobin A1c on your bloodwork. Not all doctors do that routinely, but you can always ask them to add that to the bloodwork panel to see where you are. My doctor had me do an 8 hr fast before my lab work appointment when she wanted to run an insulin resistance panel on me. If your hemoglobin A1c is at 5.2 or lower, you are good. If it's over 5.2, you better give your diet a closer look; if it's 5.7 or higher, you're heading in the wrong direction and need to get turned around.

Understanding the overlap between insulin resistance and thyroid dysfunction allows you to take targeted steps to improve your health. By addressing insulin resistance, you can support your thyroid function, boost your energy levels, and make it easier to manage your weight. Think of it as fine-tuning the machinery of your body's factory, ensuring everything runs smoothly and efficiently.

Imagine waking up every morning feeling like you've barely slept, even though you logged a full eight hours. You're dragging yourself out of bed, and no amount of coffee seems to help. This could be more than just a rough patch—welcome to the world of adrenal fatigue. Adrenal fatigue occurs when your adrenal glands, which sit atop your kidneys, can't keep up with the chronic stress you're under. These glands are responsible for producing cortisol, the hormone that helps you deal with stress. When you're constantly stressed, your adrenals work overtime, eventually leading to burnout. This condition manifests as persistent fatigue, sleep disturbances, and an overall feeling of being run down.

If you're dealing with adrenal fatigue, your thyroid might be caught in the crossfire. When your adrenals are overworked, they produce too much cortisol, which can interfere with the conversion of T4 to T3, the active form of thyroid hormone. This means your thyroid might be producing enough hormone, but your body isn't able to use it effectively. The result? You're left feeling exhausted and sluggish. Additionally, high cortisol levels can weaken your immune system, making you more susceptible to infections and even triggering autoimmune responses that can further mess with your thyroid function.

Common signs of adrenal fatigue include persistent tiredness and lack of energy, even after a good night's sleep. You might find it particularly hard to wake up in the morning feeling like you're in a perpetual state of grogginess. Cravings for salty and sugary foods are another red flag as your body tries to compensate for the lack of energy. Frequent infections and slow recovery times can also indicate that your adrenals are struggling. If you're constantly catching colds or taking forever to bounce back from minor illnesses, your adrenal health might need some attention.

Supporting your adrenal health involves a multi-faceted approach. Start with your diet. A balanced diet rich in whole foods can provide the nutrients your adrenals need to function properly. Focus on foods high in vitamin C, B vitamins, and magnesium, as these nutrients play a crucial role in adrenal health. Lean proteins, healthy fats, and complex carbohydrates can help stabilize your blood sugar levels, reducing the demand on your adrenals. Stress management is also key. Techniques like meditation and deep breathing exercises can help lower your cortisol levels, giving your adrenals a much-needed break.

Adaptogenic herbs like ashwagandha and rhodiola can be incredibly beneficial. These herbs help your body adapt to stress, reducing the impact on your adrenals. Ashwagandha, for instance, has been shown to lower cortisol levels and improve sleep quality. Rhodiola can boost your energy levels and enhance your resilience to stress. Incorporating these herbs into your routine, either through supplements or herbal teas, can support your adrenal function and, by extension, your thyroid health.

Ensuring you get enough sleep is another crucial factor. Your body does a lot of its repair work while you sleep, so aim for 7-9 hours of quality rest each night. Create a bedtime routine that promotes relaxation, like reading a book, taking a warm bath, or practicing gentle yoga. Avoid screens and caffeine in the hours leading up to bedtime to ensure a restful night's sleep. By focusing on these areas, you can support your adrenal health and improve your thyroid function, helping you feel more energized and balanced.

THE ROLE OF THE PITUITARY GLAND IN THYROID HEALTH

We will circle back to the pituitary gland to dig a little deeper on this VIP gland. Nestled snugly at the base of your brain, the pituitary gland is like the command center of your body's hormonal orchestra. This tiny, pea-sized gland sits in a bony structure called the sella turcica, and despite its small size, it wields enormous influence. The pituitary gland produces several crucial hormones, including thyroid-stimulating hormone (TSH) and adrenocorticotropic hormone (ACTH). TSH, as the name suggests, stimulates the thyroid gland to produce thyroid hormones. ACTH prompts the adrenal glands to release cortisol, the stress hormone. The pituitary's role in regulating other endocrine glands makes it the maestro of your hormonal symphony, ensuring that everything runs smoothly.

When it comes to your thyroid, the pituitary gland is the primary regulator. Think of it as the boss that tells your thyroid when to get to work. It releases TSH, which then signals the thyroid to produce and release T3 and T4. This process is part of a complex feedback loop involving the hypothalamus, pituitary, and thyroid glands. The hypothalamus releases thyrotropin-releasing hormone (TRH) when it senses that thyroid hormone levels are low. TRH then prompts the pituitary to release TSH, which stimulates the thyroid. Once the thyroid produces enough hormones, the hypothalamus and pituitary get the signal to stop releasing TRH and TSH, maintaining a delicate balance. However, when the pituitary gland malfunctions, it can throw this balance off, leading to issues like hypothyroidism or hyperthyroidism.

Pituitary gland issues can manifest in various ways. Unexplained changes in your thyroid hormone levels are a common sign. For instance, you might notice symptoms of hypothyroidism, such as fatigue and weight gain, or hyperthyroidism, like anxiety and rapid heartbeat, despite your thyroid itself being healthy. Headaches and vision problems can also indicate pituitary dysfunction, as the gland's location near the optic nerves makes it susceptible to causing these issues. Hormonal imbalances affecting other glands, such as the adrenal or reproductive glands, can further point to pituitary problems. If you're experiencing a mix of these symptoms, it's worth discussing pituitary health with your healthcare provider.

Supporting your pituitary gland involves a holistic approach. Start with a balanced diet rich in essential nutrients. Foods high in omega-3 fatty acids, like salmon and walnuts, support brain health, which is closely linked to pituitary function. B vitamins, found in leafy greens, eggs, and whole grains, are crucial for hormone production and regulation. Regular physical activity is also beneficial. Exercise increases blood flow to the brain, promoting the health of the pituitary gland. It also helps manage stress, which is important because chronic stress can negatively impact pituitary function.

Stress management techniques are another key aspect of pituitary health. Practices like meditation, deep breathing, and yoga can help lower stress levels and support overall hormonal balance. Regular medical check-ups are essential for monitoring your pituitary and thyroid health. Blood tests can help detect any imbalances early on, allowing for timely intervention. Supplements can also support pituitary health. Omega-3 fatty acids and B vitamins are particularly beneficial. These nutrients help maintain the health of the brain and endocrine system, supporting the pituitary gland's role in hormone regulation.

Focusing on these areas can support your pituitary gland and, in turn, your thyroid health. A healthy pituitary gland ensures that your hormonal orchestra plays in perfect harmony, allowing you to feel your best and maintain overall well-being.

SUPPLEMENTS: SUPPORTING YOUR THYROID NATURALLY

You might think you're eating a balanced diet, but even the best eaters can end up with nutrient deficiencies. This is especially true during periods of stress or illness when your body demands more resources to function optimally. Sometimes, no matter how many kale smoothies you gulp down, you still fall short. That's where dietary supplements come in. They can fill in the gaps, giving your thyroid the boost it needs to perform its queenly duties.

Key supplements for thyroid health include iodine, selenium, zinc, magnesium, vitamin D, and B12. Iodine is crucial for thyroid hormone production, and kelp tablets are a great natural source. Selenium acts as an antioxidant, protecting the thyroid from inflammation, while zinc and magnesium are involved in hormone production and enzyme function. Vitamin D supports immune function and overall health, and B12 helps with energy production and nerve function. Each of these supplements plays a vital role in maintaining thyroid health, ensuring that your tiny queen operates smoothly and efficiently.

Choosing high-quality supplements is key. Not all supplements are created equal, and knowing what to look for is essential. Start by reading labels for purity and potency. You want a supplement that contains what it says it does, without any unnecessary fillers or additives. Look for third-party testing and certifications, which ensure that the product has been independently verified for quality and safety. Avoid supplements with artificial colors, flavors, or preservatives. The fewer the ingredients, the better. It's like choosing a clean, organic meal over fast food—a little more effort, but so much better for you in the long run.

When it comes to supplementation protocols, one size does not fit all. A daily regimen might include a multivitamin with iodine, selenium, zinc, magnesium, vitamin D, and B12 for general thyroid support. If you have hypothyroidism, you might need higher doses of iodine and selenium. For hyperthyroidism, focus on calming the inflammation with selenium and magnesium. Timing and dosage are also crucial. Some supplements are best taken with meals, while others should be taken on an empty stomach. For instance, take iodine and selenium with your morning meal, but vitamin D can be taken with any meal that contains fat for better absorption.

Supplementation Protocols

1. General Thyroid Support: Multivitamin with iodine, selenium, zinc, magnesium, vitamin D, and B12.
2. Hypothyroidism: Higher doses of iodine and selenium.
3. Hyperthyroidism: Focus on selenium and magnesium to reduce inflammation.
4. Timing and Dosage: Iodine and selenium should be consumed with breakfast; vitamin D should be consumed with any meal containing fat.

By incorporating these supplements into your daily routine, you can naturally support your thyroid, ensuring it has all the resources it needs to function at its best. Remember, it's always a good idea to consult with a healthcare provider before starting any new supplement regimen.

As we wrap up this chapter, remember that supplements are just one piece of the puzzle in supporting your thyroid health. From balancing hormones to managing stress, every little bit helps. In the next chapter, we'll explore how diet and lifestyle choices can further enhance your thyroid function, giving your tiny queen the royal treatment she deserves.

7

CROWNING WELLNESS: LIFESTYLE CHANGES FIT FOR THE THYROID QUEEN

Imagine this: You're standing in front of the mirror, trying to muster the energy to face another day. Maybe you're feeling sluggish, your joints ache, or you're battling that stubborn weight that won't budge. What if I told you that incorporating the right kind of exercise could bring a ray of hope and relief? Yes, you heard me right! Exercise isn't just about fitting into your skinny jeans; it's about boosting your thyroid function, improving your mood, and giving you the energy to tackle life head-on.

EXERCISE AND THYROID HEALTH: THE BEST WORKOUTS FOR YOU

Regular exercise offers a plethora of benefits for your thyroid health. When you move your body, you boost your metabolism, which is the process by which your body converts what you eat and drink into energy. This is often sluggish in those with thyroid issues. Imagine your metabolism as a fire that needs kindling; exercise is the fuel that keeps it burning. Enhanced energy levels are one of the first noticeable benefits. You might start feeling more awake and less like you need a nap after every meal. Physical activity also improves your mood by releasing endorphins, the feel-good hormones. These can help reduce symptoms of depression, which are common in thyroid disorders.

Increased metabolic rate means you burn more calories, making weight management more achievable. No more feeling like you're fighting an uphill battle just to shed a few pounds. Better cardiovascular health is another perk. Like every other muscle, your heart benefits from regular exercise, reducing the risk of heart disease, which people with thyroid issues are more prone to. So, moving your body isn't just about looking good; it's about feeling good and keeping your heart healthy.

Now, let's talk about the types of exercise that are particularly beneficial for individuals with thyroid issues. Low-impact aerobic exercises, like walking and swimming, are fantastic choices. Walking is simple yet effective. A brisk 30-minute walk can work wonders for your cardiac health, sleep quality, and mental well-being. Plus, it's easy on the joints, which is a blessing if you're dealing with joint pain. Swimming and water aerobics offer a similar low-impact, full-body workout that's gentle on your joints while providing resistance to build muscle.

Strength training is another game-changer and my favorite, along with brisk walks. Building muscle mass can help boost your metabolism, making it easier to manage your weight. Women typically begin to lose muscle mass around age 30, when muscle mass and strength peak. After this point, men and women naturally experience a decline, losing about 3–5% of their muscle mass per decade, a process known as atrophy. In addition to muscle mass loss, women specifically lose strength at about 1% per year after age 35. When this muscle loss becomes more severe, it can lead to a condition called sarcopenia, which affects more than 45% of older Americans, particularly women. Sarcopenia can make daily activities like walking or standing up from a chair increasingly difficult. This decline in muscle mass and strength is caused by a combination of factors, including aging, hormonal changes, and decreased physical activity. It's super important to eat enough protein and to exercise.

Incorporate resistance training with weights or bodyweight exercises like push-ups, squats, lunges, and planks. Yoga and Pilates are excellent for flexibility and stress reduction. They strengthen and stretch your muscles and promote mindfulness and relaxation, which can help manage stress levels.

Starting and maintaining an exercise routine can feel daunting, but it doesn't have to be. Start by setting realistic goals. If you're new to exercise, aim for short, manageable sessions like a 10-minute walk or a few sets of bodyweight exercises, and gradually increase the intensity and duration. Find time in your busy schedule by breaking your workouts into shorter sessions throughout the day. Even ten minutes here and there can add up. The key is consistency over intensity. It's better to exercise regularly at a moderate pace than to push yourself too hard and risk burnout or injury.

Incorporating exercise into your daily life doesn't have to be a chore. Find activities you enjoy and make them a part of your routine. Whether it's dancing around the living room, gardening, or taking the stairs instead of the elevator, every bit of movement counts. Track your progress to stay motivated, and don't forget to celebrate your achievements, no matter how small they may seem. Exercise with a friend to make it more enjoyable and hold each other accountable.

Remember, exercise is a powerful tool in managing thyroid health, but it's essential to consult your doctor before starting any new exercise routine, especially if you have underlying health conditions. Your thyroid might be small, but with the right lifestyle changes, you can keep it reigning supreme. So, lace up those sneakers, grab your yoga mat, and get ready to give your thyroid the royal treatment it deserves.

THE IMPORTANCE OF SLEEP: RESTORING THYROID FUNCTION THROUGH REST

Let's talk about sleep, that elusive, magical state that seems harder to catch than a unicorn when you're dealing with thyroid issues. You might not realize it, but getting enough sleep is like giving your thyroid a VIP backstage pass to recovery. During sleep, your body regulates hormone production, including those crucial thyroid hormones. Imagine your body as a busy office that needs downtime to reorganize and file away important documents. Adequate sleep allows your thyroid to recalibrate and produce the hormones that keep you feeling energized and balanced.

When you're sleep-deprived, your cortisol levels shoot up. Cortisol, often dubbed the "stress hormone," can interfere with your thyroid's ability to function. I will mention again that high cortisol levels can inhibit the conversion of T4 to T3, the active form of thyroid hormone. It's like trying to run a marathon with a rock tied to your leg. You're just not going to get very far. REM sleep, the deep sleep stage where dreaming occurs, is particularly important for hormonal balance. During REM, your body performs a lot of its maintenance work, including hormone regulation. Skipping out on REM is like skipping the most important part of your thyroid's nightly to-do list.

If you're dealing with thyroid dysfunction, you're no stranger to sleep issues. Insomnia and difficulty falling asleep are common complaints. You might find yourself staring at the ceiling, counting sheep, and wondering if you'll ever drift off. Restless sleep and frequent awakenings can leave you feeling like you've been in a boxing match with your pillow. Sleep apnea, a condition where your breathing repeatedly stops and starts during sleep, is also more prevalent in individuals with thyroid issues. This can lead to severe fatigue and other health complications.

Improving your sleep quality can make a significant difference in how you feel. Start by establishing a consistent sleep schedule. Try to go to bed and wake up at the same time every day, even on weekends. This helps regulate your body's internal clock. Creating a relaxing bedtime routine can signal to your body that it's time to wind down. Think of it as easing into sleep mode. Take a warm bath, read a book, or practice some gentle stretching. Avoid stimulants like caffeine and electronics before bed. The blue light from screens can interfere with your body's production of melatonin, the hormone that regulates sleep. Aim for a dark, cool, and quiet sleep environment. Blackout curtains, a white noise machine, and a comfortable mattress can make a world of difference.

Natural sleep aids can also help you catch those Zs. Herbal teas like chamomile and passion flower have calming properties that can ease you into sleep. Melatonin supplements are another option. Melatonin is a hormone naturally produced by your body to regulate sleep-wake cycles. Taking a supplement can help if your body's production is out of whack. Essential oils like lavender and cedarwood have soothing scents that can promote relaxation. Try adding a few drops to a diffuser or spraying a bit on your pillow before bed.

Incorporating these tips into your nightly routine can improve your sleep quality and, in turn, support your thyroid health. Imagine waking up feeling refreshed, with more energy to tackle the day. It's not just a dream; it's possible with the proper sleep habits. So, as you prepare for bed tonight, remember that you're not just resting—you're giving your thyroid the royal treatment it deserves.

MIND-BODY CONNECTION: STRESS MANAGEMENT TECHNIQUES

Have you ever felt like you're juggling flaming torches while riding a unicycle on a tightrope? That's a pretty good metaphor for the kind of stress many of us deal with daily. And guess what? Your thyroid isn't a fan of this high-wire act. Chronic stress activates your body's Hypothalamic-Pituitary-Adrenal (HPA) axis, leading to increased cortisol production. While cortisol is great for short-term stress (like escaping a tiger), long-term elevated levels can mess with your thyroid hormone production and conversion. It's like your body's alarm system is stuck on "snooze," causing inflammatory processes that can further disrupt thyroid function.

One way to combat this is through mindfulness meditation and deep breathing exercises. Picture this: you're setting up a quiet space in your home, free from distractions. Sit comfortably, close your eyes, and focus on your breath. Inhale deeply through your nose, hold it for a few seconds, then exhale slowly through your mouth. Observe your thoughts without judgment. Simply notice them and let them pass like clouds in the sky. Practicing this for even just a few minutes a day can significantly reduce stress levels and help your thyroid function more smoothly.

Progressive muscle relaxation is another effective technique. Start by finding a comfortable, quiet place to sit or lie down. Begin at your toes, tensing the muscles for a few seconds, then releasing. Move up to your calves, thighs, and so on until you've tensed and relaxed every part of your body. Guided imagery can also be a fantastic stress-buster. Close your eyes and imagine a peaceful scene—a beach, a forest, or anywhere that makes you feel calm.

Visualize every detail, from the sounds to the smells, immersing yourself in the tranquility.

Yoga and Tai Chi offer a blend of physical and mental relaxation. These practices combine gentle movements with deep breathing and mindfulness, helping to lower cortisol levels and promote overall well-being. Whether it's a sun salutation in the morning or a Tai Chi session in the park, these activities can help create a sense of balance and calm.

Meet Alyssa, a mother of three who felt like she was constantly running on empty. Alyssa discovered yoga and quickly fell in love with its calming effects. She began attending classes twice a week and even practiced some poses at home. Not only did her anxiety decrease, but she also started sleeping better and felt more in control of her life. Alyssa's story is a testament to the power of combining physical movement with mental relaxation.

To get you started, here's a step-by-step guide to mindfulness meditation. Find a quiet space where you won't be disturbed. Sit down comfortably, either on a chair or the floor. Close your eyes and take a few deep breaths, inhaling through your nose and exhaling through your mouth. Focus on your breath, noticing the sensation of the air entering and leaving your body. If your mind starts to wander (and it will), gently bring your focus back to your breath. Start with just five minutes a day and gradually increase the time as you become more comfortable with the practice.

These stress management techniques are not just about reducing anxiety; they're about giving your thyroid the royal treatment it deserves. By incorporating mindfulness, progressive muscle relaxation, and yoga into your daily routine, you can help lower cortisol levels, reduce inflammation, and support your thyroid function. So, take a deep breath, find your Zen, and remember that managing stress is crucial to keeping your thyroid happy and healthy.

As we wrap up this chapter, remember that stress management, good quality sleep, and exercise are powerful ways to support your thyroid health. Your thyroid might be small, but with the right care, it can reign supremely. Next, we'll explore more in-depth of hormonal changes and perimenopause.

8

THE THYROID QUEEN'S PERIMENOPAUSAL PLAYBOOK: NAVIGATING HORMONAL CHANGES WITH GRACE

Imagine you're at a lively party, but instead of enjoying yourself, you're constantly running around trying to keep the lights on, the music playing, and the guests happy. This is what it feels like for your body during perimenopause. Hormones are the party-goers, and your thyroid is the DJ who's trying to keep everything in sync. When hormonal fluctuations hit, it's like a power surge that sends the whole party into chaos.

HORMONAL FLUCTUATIONS: THE THYROID-PERIMENOPAUSE CONNECTION

As you approach perimenopause, your body starts to produce less estrogen and progesterone, the dynamic duo of female hormones. Think of estrogen as the social butterfly and progesterone as the calm, collected friend who keeps her grounded. When these hormone levels decline, it's like the social butterfly is fluttering away, leaving the calm friend to manage the party alone. This decline doesn't happen smoothly either; it's like a roller coaster with sudden drops and unexpected twists.

During perimenopause, your hormone production becomes increasingly variable. One day, you might feel relatively normal; the next, you're hit with a wave of symptoms that make you feel anything but. This variability impacts your thyroid function because estrogen and progesterone play significant roles in how your thyroid hormones work. Estrogen influences thyroid hormone binding. It increases the production of thyroxine-binding globulin (TBG), a protein that binds to thyroid hormones in your bloodstream. When estrogen levels drop, there's less TBG, meaning more free thyroid hormones are available. It sounds good in theory, but too much free thyroid hormone can make things chaotic.

Progesterone, on the other hand, helps regulate your thyroid by supporting its function. It's like a friend who reminds you to drink water and take a break when you've had too much fun. When progesterone levels drop, your thyroid can struggle to function correctly, leading to symptoms that overlap with both peri-menopause and thyroid disorders.

Speaking of symptoms, let's talk about those delightful experiences that come with hormonal imbalances. Hot flashes are probably the most infamous. Imagine suddenly feeling like you're standing in front of a roaring bonfire, even though you're sitting in a perfectly air-conditioned room. Night sweats are the nocturnal cousin of hot flashes, soaking your sheets and leaving you feeling like you've run a marathon in your sleep. Mood swings can turn you into a roller coaster of emotions, from tears over a sappy commercial to snapping at anyone who looks at you the wrong way.

Irregular periods are another hallmark of this phase. One month, you might have a light, barely-there period, and the next, it's as if your uterus is making up for lost time with a vengeance. Heavy bleeding can be particularly concerning and exhausting, leaving you anemic and drained. These symptoms don't just make you feel miserable; they can also mimic thyroid problems, such as fatigue, weight gain, and hair loss, making it hard to figure out what's really going on.

To navigate these turbulent waters, it's crucial to monitor your hormonal changes closely. Keeping a symptom diary can be incredibly helpful. Jot down how you feel each day, noting any physical or emotional symptoms. This diary can help you spot patterns and triggers, making it easier to manage your symptoms. In the age of technology, hormone tracking apps can also be a life-saver. Apps like Clue, Flo, and MyFLO allow you to log your symptoms, track your cycle, and get insights into what's happening with your hormones.

Regular blood tests for hormone levels are another essential tool. These tests can provide a clearer picture of what's going on inside your body. They can help you and your healthcare provider make informed decisions about treatments and lifestyle changes. Ask your doctor to check your estrogen and progesterone levels along with your thyroid hormones, including TSH, free T3, free T4, and reverse T3. This monitoring process can provide reassurance and support in your health management.

The Dutch test is also another method to keep an eye on your hormones when you're feeling like your body is working against you instead of for you. The Dutch Test, which stands for Dried Urine Test for Comprehensive Hormones, works by measuring hormone metabolites and markers in urine samples to help assess hormonal health. This comprehensive test provides a detailed picture of your hormone levels and how your body is metabolizing them, which can be invaluable in understanding and managing your hormonal health.

In case you're curious, here's some bonus information.

The dutchtest.com website helps you locate providers in your area who can interpret your test results. I'll share the link and a QR code below, making it easy for you to explore this option if you're interested.

DUTCH TEST Link

Understanding the interplay between your thyroid and sex hormones during perimenopause is key to managing your health. When you know what's going on, you can take steps to support your body and keep the party (mostly) under control.

BALANCING ACT: MANAGING HORMONES AND THYROID HEALTH

Understanding the hormonal shifts of perimenopause is like mastering a complex dance routine. It's a balancing act that requires finesse and a few tricks up your sleeve. One practical approach to managing these hormonal ups and downs is through holistic methods that support your body naturally. Nutritional support is key. Think of it as giving your body the premium fuel it needs to run smoothly. Foods rich in omega-3 fatty acids, like salmon and walnuts, help reduce inflammation and support hormone health. Plenty of leafy greens, nuts, and seeds can provide the essential nutrients your body craves during this time.

Herbal remedies can also be incredibly helpful. Again, I will mention the herbs black cohosh and red clover, which have been used for centuries to balance hormones and alleviate perimenopausal symptoms. Black cohosh is particularly known for its ability to reduce hot flashes and night sweats. Red clover, on the other hand, is rich in phytoestrogens, which can help balance hormone levels naturally. Incorporating these herbs into your daily routine, whether through teas, supplements, or tinctures, can provide much-needed relief.

Lifestyle modifications play a crucial role in managing hormonal balance. As I mentioned previously, stress reduction techniques can help lower cortisol levels and support overall hormonal harmony. Sleep hygiene is another essential factor. Creating a bedtime routine that promotes relaxation can improve sleep quality, which is vital for hormonal health. Try dimming the lights an hour before bed, avoiding screens, and indulging in a warm bath or some light reading. These small changes can make a significant difference in how you feel, giving you hope and optimism for your health journey.

Hormone Replacement Therapy (HRT) is another option for managing perimenopausal symptoms, particularly for women with thyroid conditions. HRT involves taking medications that contain female hormones to replace the ones your body no longer makes. There are different types of HRT, including bioidentical hormones, which are chemically identical to those your body produces, and synthetic hormones, which are manufactured in a lab. Bioidentical hormones are often preferred by those seeking a more natural approach.

The benefits of HRT can be substantial. It can alleviate hot flashes, night sweats, mood swings, and vaginal dryness. For women with thyroid conditions, HRT can also help stabilize hormone levels, making it easier to manage thyroid symptoms. However, it's essential to weigh these benefits against potential risks. HRT can increase the risk of certain cancers, blood clots, and cardiovascular issues. Discussing these risks with your healthcare provider to determine if HRT is the right choice for you is crucial.

Integrating thyroid and hormone treatments effectively requires careful coordination with your healthcare providers. Timing and dosage adjustments for medications are necessary to ensure that both your thyroid and hormone levels remain balanced. Regular monitoring and adjusting of treatment plans are crucial to avoid potential side effects and ensure optimal health. It's like tuning a finely crafted instrument; small adjustments can make a world of difference.

Alternative therapies can also provide valuable support in managing hormone and thyroid balance. Acupuncture, for example, has been shown to regulate hormones and alleviate perimenopausal symptoms. By stimulating specific points in the body, acupuncture can help balance the flow of energy, or Qi, promoting overall well-being. Mind-body practices such as yoga and meditation can also be incredibly beneficial. These practices help reduce stress, improve mood, and support hormonal balance. Incorporating phytoestrogens and natural supplements into your routine can further support hormone health. Foods like soy, flaxseeds, and lentils are rich in phytoestrogens, which can help balance hormone levels naturally.

Navigating perimenopause with thyroid issues doesn't have to feel like an impossible task. By embracing a holistic approach, considering HRT, coordinating treatments with healthcare providers, and exploring alternative therapies, you can find the balance you need to thrive during this transitional phase.

SPECIFIC DIETARY NEEDS: NUTRITION DURING PERIMENOPAUSE

Navigating the nutritional landscape during perimenopause can feel like you're trying to read a map in a foreign language. Your body's changing needs can make it tricky to know what to eat, and hormonal fluctuations can throw your metabolism and appetite for a loop. One of the biggest challenges is the increased risk of nutrient deficiencies. As your hormones shift, your body may need more of certain nutrients to maintain balance. For example, calcium and vitamin D become crucial for bone health as estrogen levels drop, increasing the risk of osteoporosis. Meanwhile, your metabolism might slow down, making it easier to gain weight even if you're eating the same amount. Appetite changes can also be puzzling—you might find yourself craving sugary or high-carb foods, which can further mess with your blood sugar levels and overall health.

During perimenopause, maintaining a balanced diet is more important than ever. It's not just about counting calories; it's about giving your body the nutrients it needs to function optimally. Key nutrients play a significant role in supporting both thyroid and hormonal health. Calcium and vitamin D are at the top of the list for maintaining bone density and preventing fractures. As your estrogen levels decline, your bones can become more fragile, so incorporating dairy products, leafy greens, and fortified foods into your diet is essential. Omega-3 fatty acids are another powerhouse nutrient. In fatty fish like salmon and plant sources like flaxseeds and walnuts, omega-3s help reduce inflammation and support mood stability. B vitamins, including B6 and B12, are vital for energy production and stress management. They can be found in whole grains, eggs, and lean meats. Magnesium is another unsung hero. It's crucial for muscle relaxation and sleep quality, and you can find it in nuts, seeds, sweet potatoes, and dark leafy greens.

To meet these nutritional needs, focus on whole, nutrient-dense foods. Think of it as giving your body a premium fuel. Reduce your intake of processed and sugary foods, which can spike your blood sugar and leave you feeling sluggish. Instead, aim to incorporate plenty of fruits, vegetables, whole grains, and lean proteins into your meals. Phytoestrogen-rich foods like flaxseeds and soy can help balance hormone levels naturally. These plant compounds mimic estrogen in the body, providing some relief from hormonal fluctuations. Don't forget about protein; it's essential for maintaining muscle mass and supporting thyroid function. Good sources include fish, chicken, beans, and legumes.

Creating a balanced meal plan doesn't have to be complicated. Focusing on whole, nutrient-dense foods and incorporating key nutrients can support your thyroid and hormonal health during perimenopause. This approach not only helps manage symptoms but also promotes overall well-being, making this transitional phase a bit more manageable.

EMOTIONAL RESILIENCE: COPING WITH HORMONAL CHANGES

Imagine you're on an emotional roller coaster. One minute, you're on top of the world, and the next, you're plunging into the depths of despair. Hormonal changes during perimenopause can do a number on your emotional health. Fluctuations in mood and emotional stability become the new norm, leaving you feeling like you're constantly trying to catch your breath. Increased risk of anxiety and depression is also part of the package. You might find yourself worrying about things that never bothered you before or feeling a sense of dread that you can't quite shake. These emotional swings can impact your self-esteem and body image, making you question your worth and how you see yourself in the mirror.

Building emotional resilience during this time is crucial. Practicing mindfulness and meditation can help you stay grounded. Imagine finding a few quiet moments each day to sit with your thoughts, focusing on your breath and letting go of the chaos around you. It's like hitting the reset button for your mind. Engaging in regular physical activity is another way to boost your emotional resilience. Exercise releases endorphins, those feel-good hormones that can lift your mood and give you a sense of accomplishment. Whether it's a brisk walk in the park, a dance class, or a yoga session, moving your body can make a big difference.

Navigating the emotional ups and downs of perimenopause can be challenging, but with the right strategies and support, you can build emotional resilience and find your footing. Remember, it's okay to seek help and take time for yourself. You're not alone in this, and there are many tools and resources available to help you cope and thrive during this phase of life.

First and foremost, individualized treatment plans are crucial. What works for one person might not work for another, so finding a plan tailored to your specific needs is essential. Lifestyle and dietary changes play a significant role in managing symptoms and improving overall health. Incorporating nutrient-dense foods, regular exercise, and stress management techniques can make a world of difference. Persistence and self-advocacy are also vital. Navigating perimenopause and thyroid issues can be challenging, but being proactive and advocating for your health can lead to better outcomes.

In the next chapter, we'll explore the intricacies of long-term thyroid management and how to maintain your well-being through various stages of life. We'll discuss medications, alternative therapies, and the importance of ongoing support. Let's continue this journey together, ensuring your thyroid health remains a top priority.

9

ROYAL RELIEF: MEDICATIONS AND ALTERNATIVES TO SUPPORT THE THYROID QUEEN

Imagine you're at a fancy royal banquet, and the main course has just been served. But instead of a lavish feast, you're staring at a plate of plain, unseasoned tofu. That's kind of how it feels when your thyroid isn't getting the hormones it needs. Luckily, there's a solution: synthetic thyroid hormones. These tiny, miracle workers can help bring balance back to your thyroid kingdom.

SYNTHETIC THYROID HORMONES: BENEFITS AND DRAWBACKS

First up, we have Levothyroxine, the trusty foot soldier of thyroid medications. Levothyroxine is a synthetic form of the T4 hormone, and it's the most commonly prescribed thyroid medication. Think of it as a steady, reliable warrior that helps maintain your thyroid hormone levels. Levothyroxine works by replacing the T4 hormone your thyroid isn't producing enough of. The body then converts T4 into T3, the active hormone, which regulates metabolism, energy, and overall vitality.

However, like any good story, there are some plot twists. Not everyone converts T4 to T3 efficiently, which can be a challenge when using levothyroxine. This can leave you feeling like you're missing out on the full benefits, even if your TSH levels look normal on paper. You might still experience symptoms like fatigue and brain fog because your body isn't getting enough active T3. Another potential drawback is the side effects that can come with synthetic hormones. Some people report palpitations, anxiety, and insomnia, especially when they first start treatment or if their dosage is too high. It's like having a jittery jester who just won't settle down.

Next, let's talk about Liothyronine, the more dynamic knight in your thyroid army. Liothyronine is a synthetic form of the T3 hormone, and it's used when your body has trouble converting T4 to T3. This medication provides a direct boost of the active hormone, making it a powerful ally for those who need a quick pick-me-up. However, because T3 is more potent and acts faster, it's typically prescribed in smaller doses.

One of the biggest benefits of using synthetic thyroid hormones is their consistent dosage and purity. With synthetic hormones, you know exactly what you're getting every time. They're like the reliable butler who never misses a beat. This consistency makes it easier to manage your thyroid levels and ensure you're getting the exact amount of hormone you need. Synthetic hormones are also widely available and prescribed, meaning they're easy to access and have been thoroughly vetted for safety and effectiveness. Most importantly, they're effective in normalizing TSH levels, which can bring your body back into balance and alleviate many of the symptoms associated with thyroid disorders.

Absorption can also be an issue. The effectiveness of synthetic hormones can vary depending on factors like diet, other medications, and even the time of day you take your pill. It's not uncommon for some people to experience variability in how well the hormone is absorbed, leading to fluctuations in how they feel. Imagine trying to enjoy that royal banquet, but the chef keeps changing the recipe without telling you. It can be frustrating, to say the least.

To bring these points to life, let's look at Rachel's experience with levothyroxine. Rachel was diagnosed with hypothyroidism and started on levothyroxine. At first, she was relieved to finally have an answer to her debilitating fatigue and weight gain. However, she found that while her TSH levels normalized, she still felt tired and sluggish. It wasn't until her doctor added a small dose of liothyronine that she started to feel like herself again. The combination of T4 and T3 made a world of difference, bringing her energy levels back up and helping her shed those stubborn pounds.

Testimonials from others highlight both the positive outcomes and challenges of synthetic thyroid hormones. Many people find relief from their symptoms and appreciate the reliability of a consistent dosage. However, some face ongoing struggles with side effects and the fine-tuning of their treatment. It's a journey that requires patience, persistence, and a good relationship with your healthcare provider.

So, while synthetic thyroid hormones can be incredibly effective and are often the first line of treatment, they're not without their quirks. Understanding both the benefits and drawbacks can help you navigate your thyroid treatment with confidence and make informed decisions about what's best for your royal thyroid health.

NATURAL DESICCATED THYROID: AN ALTERNATIVE APPROACH

Imagine your thyroid treatment is like a wardrobe, and synthetic hormones are your reliable, go-to jeans. They work, but sometimes you crave something more tailored to your needs. Enter Natural Desiccated Thyroid (NDT), which might just be the little black dress you've been searching for. NDT is derived from porcine (pig) thyroid glands and contains a combination of T4, T3, T2, and T1 hormones. Unlike synthetic hormones that usually offer just T4 or T3, NDT provides a more holistic approach, mimicking the natural hormone production of your thyroid gland. This unique blend can be a game-changer, especially if your body struggles with converting T4 to T3.

Many patients find NDT beneficial because it more closely mimics natural thyroid hormone production. Imagine having a wardrobe that fits perfectly, no tailoring needed. That's what NDT can feel like for some people. If you have difficulty converting T4 to T3, NDT can provide that extra boost of active hormone right from the get-go. Some patients report improved symptom relief with NDT, feeling more energized and balanced. It's like having an outfit that not only looks good but feels good too, making you ready to conquer the day.

But, as with any wardrobe, there are a few considerations. NDT can be a bit like shopping from a boutique—unique but sometimes inconsistent. The potency and dosage of NDT can vary from batch to batch, which might require more frequent monitoring and adjustments. It's not always as straightforward as grabbing your usual size off the rack. Some individuals may also experience allergic reactions to the porcine-derived components, which is like discovering that your favorite fabric makes you itch. Additionally, NDT tends to be more expensive and less widely available than synthetic options, making it a bit of a splurge rather than an everyday staple.

Let's talk about Olivia's experience to illustrate this. Olivia had been on synthetic hormones for years, but despite normal lab results, she never felt quite right. She was still tired, her mood swings were unpredictable, and she couldn't shake off that brain fog. After discussing options with her doctor, she decided to switch to NDT. The transition wasn't entirely smooth—there were a few hiccups with dosage adjustments—but eventually, she found her sweet spot. Olivia noticed a significant improvement in her energy levels and mental clarity. It was like finding that perfect dress that made her feel fabulous and confident.

Testimonials from other patients also highlight the mixed bag that is NDT. Some rave about the newfound energy and sense of well-being, while others struggle with the variability and higher cost. One woman mentioned that switching to NDT was the best decision she ever made for her thyroid health, describing it as finally feeling "normal" again. Another patient, however, found the inconsistency in dosage frustrating and opted to go back to synthetic hormones. It's a bit like shopping for clothes—what works perfectly for one person might not be the best fit for another.

CUSTOMIZING YOUR TREATMENT: FINDING WHAT WORKS FOR YOU

Imagine walking into a shoe store and being handed a one-size-fits-all pair of shoes. Sounds ridiculous, right? Just like those shoes, thyroid treatments aren't one-size-fits-all. The importance of individualized treatment plans can't be overstated. Each person's thyroid journey is unique, with varying responses to medications and specific needs for dosage adjustments. What works wonders for one individual might leave another feeling just as fatigued and foggy as they did before treatment. This is why having a personalized treatment plan is crucial for effective thyroid management. Your body is unique, and it deserves a tailored approach to find the optimal balance.

Working closely with your healthcare provider is key to customizing your treatment. Start by openly communicating your symptoms and treatment goals. Don't hold back—if you're feeling off, even in ways that seem unrelated, let them know. Request comprehensive thyroid testing, including not just TSH but also Free T4, Free T3, reverse T3 and thyroid antibodies. This thorough approach can provide a clearer picture of what's happening under the hood. Regular monitoring and follow-up appointments are essential. Think of them as regular tune-ups for your thyroid, ensuring everything is running smoothly and catching any issues before they become bigger problems.

Combination therapies can be a game-changer for some people. Combining T4 and T3 medications can address the issue of poor conversion that some people face with T4-only treatments. This approach can be particularly beneficial if you're someone who doesn't feel quite right on T4 alone. Using both synthetic and natural thyroid hormones can offer a more balanced approach, providing the benefits of synthetic consistency and the holistic nature of natural hormones. Integrating medications with lifestyle changes and natural remedies can also enhance overall well-being. Incorporating stress management techniques, dietary adjustments, and supplements like selenium and zinc can complement your medication, helping you feel your best.

Adjusting your treatment plan isn't a one-and-done deal. It's an ongoing process that requires careful attention to your symptoms and lab results. Keep a symptom diary to track how you're feeling day-to-day. This can be incredibly helpful when discussing adjustments with your healthcare provider. Gradual dosage adjustments are often necessary to find the sweet spot where you feel your best. Don't be afraid to seek second opinions if you're not getting the results you need. Sometimes, a fresh perspective can make all the difference.

Take the case of Diana, who struggled with persistent fatigue and brain fog despite being on a stable dose of levothyroxine. After discussing her symptoms with her doctor, they decided to add a small dose of liothyronine to her regimen. The change wasn't immediate, but over a few weeks, Dianna began to notice a significant improvement in her energy levels and mental clarity. She kept a detailed symptom diary, which helped her doctor make precise adjustments to her dosage. This collaborative approach allowed Dianna to find a treatment plan that truly worked for her.

Let's not forget the importance of regular check-ins with your healthcare provider. These appointments are crucial for monitoring your progress and making necessary adjustments. They're like pit stops in a long race, ensuring that everything is functioning optimally. At each visit, bring your symptom diary and any questions or concerns you have. This proactive approach ensures that you're an active participant in your treatment plan, working in partnership with your healthcare provider to achieve the best possible outcomes.

Customizing your thyroid treatment is like finding the perfect recipe. It requires the right ingredients, careful adjustments, and a bit of patience. But when you get it right, the results can be life-changing.

COMBINING MEDICATIONS WITH NATURAL REMEDIES: A BALANCED APPROACH

Imagine you're an artist, and your thyroid health is the masterpiece you're working on. Sometimes, using just one type of brush isn't enough to create the detailed, vibrant picture you envision. Combining medications with natural remedies can be like adding different brush strokes to enhance your painting. This balanced approach can offer enhanced symptom relief and improved overall well-being by addressing both the root causes and symptoms of thyroid issues.

Combining medications with natural remedies brings together the best of both worlds. Medications like levothyroxine can stabilize your hormone levels, while natural remedies can address underlying issues like inflammation and stress. Think of it as adding a touch of vibrant color to your steady base coat, creating a fuller, more balanced picture of health. Herbal supplements like ashwagandha and rhodiola can help manage stress, which is known to impact thyroid function. These adaptogens are like your personal stress-relievers, helping your body cope with daily pressures that can otherwise throw your thyroid off balance. Nutritional support is another critical component. Supplements like selenium, zinc, and iodine can provide the building blocks your thyroid needs to function optimally. Selenium, for instance, helps convert T4 to T3, the active form of thyroid hormone, making it easier for your body to use. Zinc plays a role in hormone production, while iodine is essential for thyroid hormone synthesis. Incorporating these nutrients can be as simple as adding a handful of Brazil nuts to your diet for selenium or enjoying seafood rich in iodine.

However, it's essential to monitor and adjust both medications and natural remedies carefully. Regular lab tests and symptom tracking are your tools for ensuring everything is working as it should.

Keep a health journal where you note down how you feel each day, any new symptoms, and your energy levels. This helps you and your healthcare provider make informed decisions about your treatment. Communicate any changes you notice with your healthcare provider. If you start feeling jittery or notice new symptoms, it might be time to adjust your dosages or try a different supplement. Adjusting dosages and remedies as needed ensures that your treatment remains effective and tailored to your evolving needs.

Take Mia's experience as a case in point. Mia struggled with hypothyroidism and found that while levothyroxine helped, she still felt fatigued and foggy. After researching and consulting with her doctor, she started incorporating natural remedies like ashwagandha for stress and selenium for thyroid support. Over time, she noticed a significant improvement in her energy levels and mental clarity. Her experience highlights the potential benefits of a combined approach. Testimonials from others also underscore the positive outcomes of integrating medications with natural remedies. Many people report feeling more balanced and energetic when they combine the two approaches. One woman mentioned that adding rhodiola to her routine helped her manage stress better, which in turn improved her thyroid function. Another patient found that incorporating iodine-rich foods made a noticeable difference in her overall well-being. However, it's not always a smooth journey. Some people face challenges, like finding the right combination of supplements or dealing with initial side effects. It's essential to approach this process with patience and flexibility, knowing that adjustments might be necessary along the way.

Combining medications with natural remedies offers a holistic approach to thyroid health. By addressing both the root causes and symptoms, you can achieve enhanced symptom relief and improved overall well-being. Just like an artist uses different brushes to create a masterpiece, integrating various treatments can help you achieve a balanced, vibrant picture of health.

LONG-TERM MEDICATION: IS IT NECESSARY?

Let's tackle the big question: Is long-term medication necessary for managing thyroid conditions? This isn't a one-size-fits-all answer. The necessity often hinges on several factors, such as the severity and type of thyroid condition you're dealing with. For instance, someone with severe hypothyroidism may require life-long medication to maintain stable hormone levels, while someone with a milder form might manage with intermittent treatment. Your response to initial treatment also plays a crucial role. If you find that your symptoms are well-controlled and your thyroid levels remain stable with medication, long-term use might be the best option. However, if you're experiencing side effects or inconsistent results, it might be worth exploring other avenues. Underlying causes and risk factors, such as autoimmune conditions like Hashimoto's thyroiditis, can also dictate the need for ongoing medication.

Long-term medication can offer significant benefits, including stable hormone levels and effective symptom management. Imagine finally being able to get through the day without needing a nap or feeling like you're wading through quicksand. That's the kind of stability long-term medication can bring. However, it's not all rainbows and unicorns. There are potential risks to consider, such as side effects that can vary from mild (like occasional headaches) to more severe (like palpitations or anxiety). Dependency on medication is another concern. Once you start, you may need to continue to maintain your thyroid levels, which isn't always a bad thing but is something to be aware of. There's also the cost factor—those little pills can add up over time, hitting your wallet harder than you might expect.

So, what if you're not keen on the idea of taking medication forever? There are alternative strategies for long-term thyroid health management. Lifestyle and dietary changes can make a huge difference. For example, incorporating a diet rich in selenium, zinc, and iodine can support thyroid function naturally. Regular exercise and stress management techniques like yoga or mindfulness can also help maintain your thyroid health. Regular monitoring and preventive measures are crucial. Keeping an eye on your thyroid levels through periodic testing can help catch any imbalances early, allowing for timely adjustments. Natural and holistic approaches, such as herbal supplements or acupuncture, can also complement these efforts. These alternatives might not completely replace the need for medication, but they can certainly enhance your overall well-being and possibly reduce your dependency on pharmaceuticals.

Lydia's journey with lifelong thyroid medication offers valuable insights. Diagnosed with hypothyroidism in her twenties, she started on levothyroxine and found it incredibly effective. Over the years, she's had to tweak her dosage and incorporate lifestyle changes like a thyroid-friendly diet and regular exercise. Despite some ups and downs, Lydia has managed to live a full, active life. She emphasizes the importance of finding a supportive healthcare provider and being proactive about her health. Testimonials from others highlight both the benefits and challenges of long-term medication. One woman mentioned that while the medication stabilized her symptoms, she had to deal with side effects like occasional anxiety and insomnia. Another patient found that a combination of medication and lifestyle changes allowed her to reduce her dosage over time, achieving a balanced approach that worked for her.

Assessing the need for long-term medication is a nuanced process that involves considering the severity of your condition, your response to treatment, and underlying risk factors. While long-term medication can offer stability and symptom relief, it's essential to be aware of potential side effects and costs. Exploring alternative strategies, such as lifestyle changes and natural remedies, can provide additional support and potentially reduce your dependency on medication. By staying informed and working closely with your healthcare provider, you can find the best approach to manage your thyroid health effectively.

As we wrap up this chapter, remember that the journey to optimal thyroid health is personal and unique. Whether through long-term medication, lifestyle changes, or a combination of both, finding what works best for you is key. Next, we'll explore the importance of ongoing education and support systems to keep you informed and motivated on your path to thyroid wellness.

10

THE QUEEN'S REIGN: LONG-TERM MANAGEMENT AND EMPOWERMENT FOR HER HEALTH

Imagine you're a queen overseeing a bustling kingdom. Your thyroid is the command center, ensuring everything runs smoothly. But what happens when this command center falters? The answer lies in finding the right balance of medications to restore order and keep your kingdom thriving. Let's explore the different types of thyroid medications and how to manage them effectively.

Reflection Section: Medication Management Checklist

1. Regular Blood Tests: Schedule tests every 3-6 months to monitor TSH, Free T3, Reverse T3, and Free T4 levels.
2. Consistent Timing: Take your medication at the same time each day, preferably on an empty stomach.
3. Avoid Interfering Substances: Keep a gap of at least four hours between your medication and calcium or iron supplements.
4. Symptom Tracking: Keep a journal to note any changes in

symptoms and discuss them with your healthcare provider.

5. Open Communication: Maintain regular check-ins with your healthcare provider to adjust dosages as needed.

Managing thyroid medications effectively requires a combination of the right treatment, regular monitoring, and open communication with your healthcare provider. By paying attention to your body's signals and making necessary adjustments, you can maintain balance and ensure your thyroid kingdom thrives.

CAN THE THYROID BE RESTORED? EXPLORING THE POSSIBILITIES

The concept of thyroid regeneration might sound like something out of a sci-fi movie, but it's a topic that's gaining traction in the medical community. Scientific studies have shown that thyroid cells have some potential for regeneration, although it's not as straightforward as flipping a switch. Researchers are exploring the ability of thyroid cells to regenerate and repair, which could mean a future where thyroid dysfunction is less of a lifelong sentence. Stem cell therapy is one of the most exciting areas of research. Imagine stem cells as tiny, magical workers that can transform into various types of cells, including thyroid cells. While this research is still in its early stages, the potential for stem cell therapy to restore thyroid function is promising. However, it's essential to remember that these advancements are not yet widely available and still under rigorous study. So, while thyroid regeneration is thrilling, it's not a guaranteed solution yet.

Medical advancements are also paving the way for potential future treatments in thyroid restoration. Regenerative medicine is rapidly evolving, with researchers exploring various methods to repair and regenerate damaged tissues. This includes not only stem cell therapy but also gene editing and other innovative techniques. Clinical trials are ongoing, and while we're not quite there yet, the future looks promising. Staying informed about these advancements is crucial. Keep an eye on new research and clinical trials, and consult with medical professionals knowledgeable about these emerging therapies. They can provide guidance on the latest treatments and help you make informed decisions about your health, empowering you to take control of your health journey.

In summary, while thyroid regeneration is still in its early stages, you can support your thyroid naturally in several ways. A nutrient-dense diet, targeted supplements, and herbal remedies can all help promote thyroid health. Real-life examples show that lifestyle changes can lead to significant improvements, and ongoing research in regenerative medicine offers hope for the future. Staying informed and working closely with your healthcare provider can help you take advantage of these advancements and support your thyroid health effectively.

LIVING YOUR BEST LIFE: EMPOWERMENT AND LONG-TERM WELLNESS

Balance is vital to living your best life with thyroid disease or during perimenopause. Picture it like a three-legged stool: physical health, emotional well-being, and mental clarity. If one leg is wobbly, the whole thing tips over. That's why a holistic approach to wellness, considering all aspects of your health, is so important.

Be sure to stay grounded and manage stress, which, as you know, can wreak havoc on your thyroid. Start with just five minutes a day. Sit in a quiet space, close your eyes, and focus on your breath. It might feel strange at first, but over time, this can become a sanctuary from the chaos of daily life. Another great addition to your routine is regular physical activity. This doesn't mean you need to run a marathon; even a brisk walk can do wonders. Tailor your exercise routine to your needs and listen to your body. Some days, yoga might be more your speed, while other days, you might feel up for a more intense workout.

Prioritizing mental health and stress management is crucial. Life can throw curveballs, and how you handle them can make all the difference. Find what works for you—whether it's talking to a therapist, journaling, or simply taking time to relax with a good book. The goal is to create a toolkit of strategies that help you stay resilient and optimistic.

Maintaining motivation and consistency in your wellness journey can be challenging, so setting realistic, achievable goals is important. Break them down into smaller steps, and celebrate each milestone. Did you manage to meditate every day this week? That's a win! Treat yourself to something small, like a new book or a relaxing bath. Creating a support system is also vital. Surround yourself with friends, family, and healthcare providers who understand your struggles and cheer you on. They can offer encouragement, hold you accountable, and provide a shoulder to lean on when things get tough.

Let's not underestimate the power of community and support networks. Engaging with supportive communities can provide a sense of belonging and understanding that's hard to find elsewhere. Consider joining thyroid support groups or forums where you can share experiences and gain insights from others on a similar path, fostering a sense of connection and understanding.

Here's a final nugget of wisdom: long-term wellness is not about perfection but about progress. It's about making small, consistent changes that add up over time. It's about being kind to yourself, recognizing your efforts, and understanding that setbacks are part of the process. Keep your eyes on the big picture and remember that every step you take is a step toward a healthier, happier you. Set expectations for yourself up front; know that it could take longer than you would like to make these lifestyle changes, but don't beat yourself up either if you fall off the course. Just get back on track when you're ready to tackle the challenges of lifestyle changes. Don't give up on yourself and chase that vitality of health that you know you can have; it's just a matter of finding the right Doctor to work with you on your health journey.

PODCASTS AND BOOKS FOR CONTINUED LEARNING

Imagine you're at a bookstore, surrounded by a treasure trove of knowledge. Each book is a key to understanding a new facet of thyroid health. Now, think of podcasts as your portable bookstore, offering wisdom right into your ears as you go about your day. Additionally, gaining deeper insights into thyroid function helps you understand what your body is going through. It's like being given a map in a maze. You'll know why you're feeling the way you do, which can be empowering and reassuring. This knowledge enables you to have more meaningful conversations with your healthcare providers, ensuring you get the best care possible.

Moreover, finding new strategies for managing symptoms can be a game-changer. Maybe you'll discover a new dietary tweak, a supplement you hadn't considered, or a stress management technique that works wonders for you. These minor adjustments can add up to significant improvements in your quality of life. Staying motivated and inspired is crucial, too. Hearing success stories or learning about the latest breakthroughs can give you hope and keep you committed to your health journey.

One of the easiest ways to stay informed and inspired is by tuning into podcasts. They're like having a health coach in your pocket. Here are some highly recommended ones. "The Thyroid Fixer" by Dr. Amie Hornaman is fantastic. I recently discovered her from another health podcast that I listen to. Dr. Amie dives deep into various thyroid issues, offering practical advice and sharing real-life success stories. Her episodes are packed with valuable insights, making complex topics easy to understand. Another great listen is the "The Resetter Podcast" by Dr. Mindy Pelz. While it covers a broad range of health topics, there are numerous episodes dedicated to thyroid health. Mindy's style makes it feel like you're chatting with a friend, and her interviews with experts provide a wealth of information.

Then there is "The Dr. Axe Show" by Dr. Josh Axe, a must-listen. Dr. Axe combines conventional medicine with natural remedies, offering a balanced perspective on thyroid health. His episodes cover everything from diet and supplements to stress management and exercise. Then there's "Thyroid Nation RADIO" by Danna Bowman and Tiffany Mladinich. This podcast is explicitly tailored for thyroid patients, offering support, education, and inspiration. Danna and Tiffany's passion for thyroid advocacy shines through in every episode, making it both informative and uplifting.

Incorporating ongoing education into your routine doesn't have to be overwhelming. It can be as simple as listening to a podcast during your morning commute or reading a chapter of a book before bed. The key is to make it a habit, a part of your daily life. The more you learn, the more empowered you'll feel to take control of your health. You'll be better equipped to make informed decisions, advocate for yourself, and confidently explore new treatment options.

So, keep that curiosity alive. Embrace the role of a lifelong learner. Your health is a dynamic, ever-evolving journey; staying informed is your best tool for navigating it. Remember, knowledge is power, and the more you know about your thyroid health, the better you can manage it. Keep tuning in, keep reading, and keep growing. Your thyroid—and your overall well-being—will thank you.

CONCLUSION

Wow, what a journey we've had together! We've traversed the intricate world of thyroid health, from understanding the basics to diving deep into hormones, natural remedies, and lifestyle changes. It's been a ride full of discoveries, a few "aha" moments, and hopefully, a lot of laughs and learning.

Let's quickly recap what we've covered. We started by meeting your tiny yet mighty thyroid queen, understanding her role, and how she rules over your metabolism and energy levels. We then explored the various hormones she produces and how they affect your body. From there, we delved into the common disorders like hypothyroidism and hyperthyroidism, Hashimoto's, and Graves' disease, and discussed their symptoms and treatments. Along the way, we didn't shy away from the invisible triggers like environmental toxins and viral infections that can wreak havoc on your thyroid.

We then ventured into the realm of hormonal imbalances, especially as they relate to perimenopause—a time when many of you might feel like your body has its own agenda. We didn't stop there;

we also tackled the importance of gut health, the impact of stress, and how things like insulin resistance and adrenal fatigue can complicate the thyroid picture even further.

One of our significant stops was understanding your thyroid blood panel. Armed with this knowledge, you can now better engage with your healthcare provider and ensure your symptoms aren't being dismissed. We also explored natural remedies, dietary changes, and the importance of gut and pituitary health in supporting your thyroid queen. And let's not forget the nitty-gritty of medications and the potential for thyroid regeneration.

So, what are the key takeaways? Here's a quick rundown:

- Your thyroid is the queen of your metabolism and plays a crucial role in your overall health.
- Understanding thyroid hormones (T4, T3, and Reverse T3) and their balance can help you grasp why you feel the way you do.
- Common thyroid disorders have distinct symptoms but often overlap, making accurate diagnosis essential.
- Environmental toxins, stress, and hormonal changes can significantly impact thyroid function.
- A balanced diet rich in iodine, selenium, and other nutrients can support thyroid health.
- Regular monitoring of your thyroid levels and understanding your blood panel can help you stay proactive.
- Natural remedies, lifestyle changes, and proper medication can all work together for optimal health.
- Never underestimate the importance of gut health and its connection to your thyroid.
- Exercise and stress management are essential to thyroid health.

Now, it's your turn to take action. Your journey to better thyroid health doesn't end here—it's just beginning. Start by making small, manageable changes in your diet, incorporating stress-reducing activities like yoga or meditation, and being proactive about your health. Schedule regular check-ups and blood tests, and don't hesitate to seek second opinions if something doesn't feel right. Advocate for yourself. Your health is worth it!

Remember, you are not alone in this journey. There are communities, support groups, and healthcare providers who can offer guidance and support. Share your experiences, learn from others, and keep pushing forward. Knowledge is power, and now you have the tools to manage your thyroid health effectively.

Let's bring it home with this: Living with thyroid issues or navigating perimenopause can feel like an uphill battle, but with the correct information and support, you are more than capable of reclaiming your health and vitality. Take it one step at a time, celebrate your progress, and trust that brighter days are ahead.

Thank you for joining me on this journey. I hope you found this book informative, engaging, and empowering. Your thyroid may be small, but with the proper care, she can indeed be mighty. Here's to your health, energy, and the wonderful life that awaits you. You've got this!

REFERENCES

The thyroid gland in ancient Greece: a historical perspective https://link.springer.com/article/10.1007/s42000-018-0039-z

Thyroid Hormone Regulation of Metabolism - PMC https://www.ncbi.nlm.nih.gov/pmc/articles/PMC4044302/

Hypothyroidism vs. Hyperthyroidism - Verywell Health https://www.verywellhealth.com/hypothyroidism-hyperthyroidism-5180646

Environmental Issues in Thyroid Diseases - PMC https://www.ncbi.nlm.nih.gov/pmc/articles/PMC5357628/

Hashimoto's disease: MedlinePlus Genetics https://medlineplus.gov/genetics/condition/hashimotos-disease/

Understanding the Role of Cortisol in Thyroid Function ... https://www.rupahealth.com/post/the-stress-thyroid-link-understanding-the-role-of-cortisol-in-thyroid-function-within-functional-medicine

Efficacy of the Autoimmune Protocol Diet as Part of a Multi- ... https://www.ncbi.nlm.nih.gov/pmc/articles/PMC6592837/

Thyroid Disrupting Chemicals - PMC https://www.ncbi.nlm.nih.gov/pmc/articles/PMC5751186/

Hypothyroidism | Nature Reviews Disease Primers https://www.nature.com/articles/s41572-022-00357-7

Hyperthyroidism - Symptoms and causes https://www.mayoclinic.org/diseases-conditions/hyperthyroidism/symptoms-causes/syc-20373659

Hashimoto Thyroiditis - StatPearls https://www.ncbi.nlm.nih.gov/books/NBK459262/

Graves' disease - Symptoms and causes https://www.mayoclinic.org/diseases-conditions/graves-disease/symptoms-causes/syc-20356240

Thyroid Blood Test: Types, Normal Levels, Analyzing Results https://www.verywellhealth.com/interpret-your-thyroid-test-results-3231840

Pitfalls in the measurement and interpretation of thyroid ... - NCBI https://www.ncbi.nlm.nih.gov/pmc/articles/PMC3857600/

Best At-Home Thyroid Test | Our Top Choices of 2024 https://www.innerbody.com/home-health-tests/home-thyroid-test

How to Find the Best Healthcare Providers for Thyroid Care https://www.verywellhealth.com/find-best-doctors-for-thyroid-care-3232861

Hashimoto's and Leaky Gut - What is the Connection? https://www.thyforlife.com/hashimotos-and-leaky-gut/

Thyroid-Gut-Axis: How Does the Microbiota Influence ... https://www.ncbi.nlm.nih.gov/pmc/articles/PMC7353203/

Effect of probiotics or prebiotics on thyroid function: A meta- ... https://journals.plos.org/plosone/article?id=10.1371/journal.pone.0296733

Digestive Enzymes and Thyroid Health https://www.naturalendocrinesolutions.com/articles/digestive-enzymes-thyroid-health/

Endocrine System: What It Is, Function, Organs & Diseases https://my.clevelandclinic.org/health/body/21201-endocrine-system

Role of Estrogen in Thyroid Function and Growth Regulation https://www.ncbi.nlm.nih.gov/pmc/articles/PMC3113168/

Perimenopause and Thyroid Problems—common and ... https://www.cemcor.ubc.ca/ask/perimenopause-and-thyroid-problems-common-and-confusing

Supplements and Thyroid Health: What to Know https://www.healthline.com/nutrition/thyroid-vitamins

Best exercises for hypothyroidism: How staying active can ... https://www.medicalnewstoday.com/articles/best-exercises-for-hypothryoidism

Thyroid Dysfunction and Sleep Disorders - PMC https://www.ncbi.nlm.nih.gov/pmc/articles/PMC8423342/

Stress Management in Women with Hashimoto's thyroiditis https://www.ncbi.nlm.nih.gov/pmc/articles/PMC6688766/

5 Ways to Gently Detox for Better Thyroid Function https://www.restartmed.com/thyroid-detox/?srsltid=AfmBOopYR7fifYBkqAJWOBKtoiGQEnWMiZMSwhb56T5I5gEoK2sgO1VI

Thyroid Dysfunction in Peri-and Postmenopausal Women ... https://www.ncbi.nlm.nih.gov/pmc/articles/PMC10398375/

Role of Estrogen in Thyroid Function and Growth Regulation https://www.ncbi.nlm.nih.gov/pmc/articles/PMC3113168/

10 Natural Ways to Balance Your Hormones - Healthline https://www.healthline.com/nutrition/balance-hormones

Sluggish Thyroid? How to Eat for Optimal Support & Energy https://drannagarrett.com/sluggish-thyroid-how-to-eat-for-optimal-support-energy/

Use of Combination of Oral Levothyroxine and Liothyronine in ... https://www.ncbi.nlm.nih.gov/pmc/articles/PMC9758553

Desiccated thyroid extract vs Levothyroxine in the ... https://www.thyroid.org/patient-thyroid-information/ct-for-patients/vol-6-issue-8/vol-6-issue-8-p-3/

Natural treatments and home remedies for hypothyroidism https://www.medicalnewstoday.com/articles/remedies-for-hypothyroidism

Adverse effects of long-term Levothyroxine therapy in ... https://www.ncbi.nlm.nih.gov/pmc/articles/PMC9052136/

Use of Combination of Oral Levothyroxine and Liothyronine in ... https://www.ncbi.nlm.nih.gov/pmc/articles/PMC9758553

Natural Desiccated Thyroid Medication: Fact and Fiction https://www.palomahealth.com/learn/natural-desiccated-thyroid-medication?srsltid=AfmBOoqLatQ8g687v7Bgd7et-LWJySO2ogU3Y_aj88S6Sk2CQNMlh1Ev

Thymus Degeneration and Regeneration – PMC https://www.ncbi.nlm.nih.gov/pmc/articles/PMC8442952/

Hashimoto Diet: Overview, Foods, Supplements, and Tips https://www.healthline.com/nutrition/hashimoto-diet

Brennan, F. (2023, June 12). *Member Listings: SMART Member.* IAOMT. https://iaomt.org/member-listings-smart-member/?utm_medium&utm_source&utm_campaign=s.m.a.r.t+choice+dentist+directory+%28safe+amalgam++removal%29

Society, E. (2022, August 11). *Endocrine-Disrupting chemicals (EDCs).* Endocrine Society. https://www.endocrine.org/patient-engagement/endocrine-library/edcs

Thyroid antibodies explained. (n.d.). British Thyroid Foundation. https://www.btf-thyroid.org/thyroid-antibodies-explained